ECCENTRIC MUSCLE TRAINING IN SPORTS AND ORTHOPAEDICS

10/16/93

To Patty,

Best wishes in your practice!

Enjoy the book!

ECCENTRIC MUSCLE TRAINING IN SPORTS AND ORTHOPAEDICS

Mark Albert, M.Ed., P.T., A.T.C.

Instructor, Department of Physical Therapy
Georgia State University
Physical Therapist and Athletic Trainer
Georgia Tech Athletic Association
Private Practice
Atlanta, Georgia

CHURCHILL LIVINGSTONE
New York, Edinburgh, London, Melbourne, Tokyo

Library of Congress Cataloging-in-Publication Data

Albert, Mark.
Eccentric muscle training in sports and orthopaedics / Mark Albert.
p. cm.
Includes bibliographical references (p.) and index.
ISBN 0-443-08754-7
1. Exercise therapy. 2. Weight training. 3. Exercise--Physiological aspects.a. I. Title.
RM725.A43 1991
615.8′2—dc20 90-26175
CIP

Distributed in the United Kingdom by Churchill Livingstone, Robert Stevenson House, 1–3 Baxter's Place, Leith Walk, Edinburgh EH1 3AF, and by associated companies, branches, and representatives throughout the world.

Acquisitions Editor: *Kim Loretucci*
Copy Editor: *David Terry*
Production Designer: *Angela Cirnigliaro*
Production Supervisor: *Jeanine Furino*

Printed in the United States of America

First published in 1991 7 6 5 4 3 2 1

To my parents, Lloyd and Donna, and to Clella, whose love and patience have streamlined the process

Contributors

Mark Albert, M.Ed., P.T., A.T.C.
Instructor, Department of Physical Therapy, Georgia State University; Physical Therapist and Athletic Trainer, Georgia Tech Athletic Association; Private Practice, Atlanta, Georgia

Peter Draovitch, M.S., A.T.C., P.T., C.S.C.S.
Director of Sports Therapy Services, Physical Therapy Specialists of the Palm Beaches, Palm Beach Gardens, Florida

Patricia A. Hageman, M.S., P.T.
Assistant Professor and Director, Division of Physical Therapy Education, University of Nebraska College of Medicine, Omaha, Nebraska

Jim Lathrop, M.Ed., C.S.C.S.
Director of Player Development, Georgia Tech Athletic Association, Atlanta, Georgia

Teresa A. Sorensen, P.T.
Clinical Supervisor, Midwest Sports and Industrial Rehabilitation, Omaha, Nebraska

Michael L. Voight, M.Ed., P.T., A.T.C., C.S.C.S.
Instructor, Department of Orthopaedics and Rehabilitation, Division of Physical Therapy, University of Miami School of Medicine, Coral Gables, Florida; Director, S.T.A.R. Sports Medicine Center, North Miami, Florida

Foreword

It is indeed an honor and a privilege to be invited to write the foreword to this interesting and timely book on eccentric muscle training. In writing this, I realized that I have been working clinically with eccentrics for approximately 20 years. Initially, my experiences with eccentric exercises were in developing sports preventive/conditioning programs and rehabilitation programs. During the last 7 years, since the advent of eccentric isokinetics (which has allowed for better control of variables and more objective documentation), I have also been involved in numerous research projects. Although mistakes in the clinic have been made, we have also learned from those mistakes. Perhaps these experiences enable me to share some of my comments with you and to offer my support to the author of this book.

Periodically, there have been trends and "buzzwords" that have pervaded the sports and orthopaedics physical therapy profession: mobilization, isokinetics, muscle, myofascial release techniques, open/closed kinetic chain activities, and now eccentrics and plyometrics. Many of these trends are initially based on empirical findings and lack the scientific documentation required to establish their validity and longevity in clinical practice. Over time, however, their value is demonstrated through research and documentation. At this point, virtually all clinicians treating sports and orthopaedic injuries have incorporated some aspect of eccentric muscle training into their rehabilitation and conditioning programs. Thus, the need for an initial book that provides the most efficient implementation and integration of this exercise mode, as this one does, is obvious.

The explosion of information on muscle training with concentric exercise and concentric isokinetics in the 1980s makes this publication on eccentrics a very timely one. Much remains to be learned in the 1990s: certainly our knowledge in the area of eccentric muscle training, using isotonics, isokinetics, plyometrics, impulse inertial exercise, and new forms of exercise (that we may not even be aware of at the present time) needs to be expanded. Fortunately, with the more recent introduction of computerized eccentric instrumentation, we are now able to control more variables as well as improve the computerized objective documentation in eccentric training. Therefore, this book is by no means the "final word" on eccentrics, but the beginning of the development of a new and exciting body of knowledge. I think the editor and contributors would agree with me on this point.

My advice to you: read the book to learn and share information from it; think, question, and evaluate the information; keep an open mind about the content; but most of all, use it to improve the quality and diversity of patient care.

George J. Davies, M.Ed., P.T., A.T.C.
Associate Professor, Department of Physical Therapy
University of Wisconsin School of Health and Human Sciences
Lacrosse, Wisconsin

Preface

This book describes and illustrates the scientific and clinical rationale for eccentric muscle training from the perspectives of literature, functional importance, and clinical experience. We focus on the principles and guidelines that enable the exercise specialist to safely and effectively apply eccentric muscle loads, regardless of the particular patient problem, treatment goal, or available equipment. Through this book we hope to make the clinician more sensitive to the clinical question, "Is this particular patient's problem being caused by inability to produce appropriate muscle tension in a specific mode of contraction (i.e., eccentric)?"

Functional eccentric muscle training is classified and addressed in the following five areas:

1. General principles—isotonics, including hand-held weights and machines, and functional, daily demands (Chs. 1, 2, and 3)
2. Plyometrics—a system of training developed in Eastern Europe and the Soviet Union (Ch. 4)
3. Inertial loading—a new form of muscle training introduced in 1985 (Ch. 5)
4. Isokinetics—applied through the use of robotics (Ch. 6)
5. Free weights and power lifting—specifics of weights for explosive muscular performance (Ch. 7)

It is my sincere hope that this initial effort to synthesize clinical perspectives with scientific principles of eccentric muscle loading will serve as a stimulus to promote research and thereby advance our current knowledge and practice. The book can be used by educators to present the principles to their students, by investigators to pose questions for experimental or clinical research, and by clinicians in various disciplines as a guide to increased and improved patterns of practice. Ultimately, precise documentation and clinical studies will produce a growth in the use and applications of eccentric training. This in turn, we believe, will result in improved and diversified patient care.

Mark Albert, M.Ed., P.T., A.T.C

Contents

1

Introduction

DESCRIPTION OF ECCENTRIC MUSCLE CONTRACTION

In the past few years, no other aspect of muscle loading (specific stress applied to the musculotendinous unit) has been described, discussed, or investigated in the literature more than eccentrics. For the purposes of this book, *eccentrics* will be defined as . . . a type of muscle loading that involves an external force application with resultant tension increase during physical lengthening of the musculotendinous unit. The surge of interest in this area has produced a clear departure from previous clinical thought that regarded eccentrics as merely the return or second phase of isotonics. Indeed, isotonic loading does consist of two distinct phases, concentrics and eccentrics; each possesses a number of separate and unique physiologic properties and, consequently, each has a markedly different potential for training effects. Common clinical and functional synonyms for eccentric exercise are numerous (Table 1-1).

Due to the recognized multiple functions of muscle (skeletal motor, stabilizer, and shock absorber[1] and its highly mutable (or plastic) nature, better awareness of muscle biology, with emphasis on areas such as eccentrics, will assist the clinician in providing skilled, progressive health care programs. Hence, concepts of muscle biology provide the scientific basis for improved clinical practice methods and the design of innovative approaches to patient care and performance training.[2]

The rapid movement toward specialization within the health science professions has produced increased reliance on sophisticated equipment, continual growth of the knowledge base of therapeutic exercise, and an emerging emphasis on clinical, field, and experimental research regarding the effects of exercise on the musculoskeletal, neuromuscular, and cardiovascular systems. Clearly, the appropriate application of research to clinical and sports training settings will power the growth and evolution of exercise training into the next decade.

Technologic growth has provided the parallel fields of physical therapy, sports medicine, and rehabilitation with promising new exercise equipment for muscle training. Subsequent new biomechanical designs in conjunction with ergonomic principles and specialized materials have improved the potential for optimal muscle training.

As in all biomedical equipment areas, the diversity of equipment lines has increased dramatically, while the pioneer standard systems (Cybex and Nautilus) now face a host of competitive alternatives in the marketplace (Table 1-2).

Table 1-1. Synonyms for Eccentric Loading

Clinical	Functional
Negative work	Descending (stairs, ramps, sitting) (Fig. 1-2)
Negatives	Lowering (objects, body)
Deceleration (Fig. 1-1)	Landing (from jump. fall) (Fig. 1-3)
Shock absorbers	Restraining (dog on a leash) (Fig. 1-4)

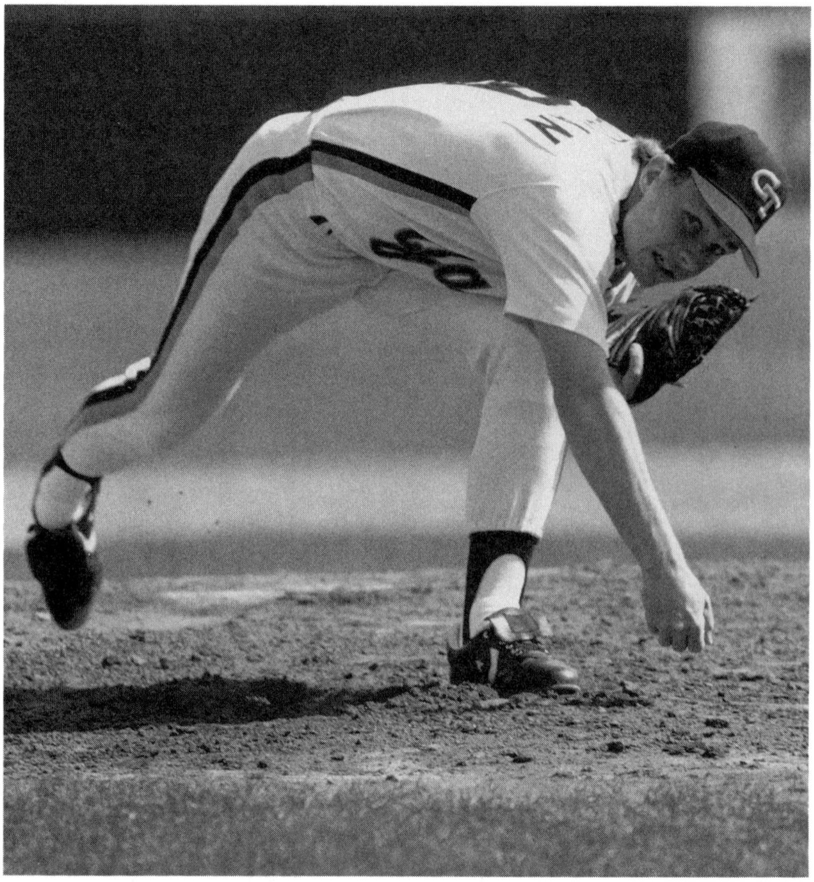

Fig. 1-1. Example of deceleration (end of follow-through phase of a baseball pitch).

RATIONALE FOR ECCENTRIC TRAINING

Since 1982, the introduction of isokinetic dynamometers with eccentric loading capacity has inspired interest in the clinical use of eccentric training and has provided a reliable method of conducting research into the specific physiologic effects of eccentric training (see Ch. 2). New perspectives presented in the professional literature have increased awareness of specific therapeutic and performance protocols that have promising, but largely unverified, potential. Clinical use of any of the multiple exercise systems that provide an eccentric component (Table 1-2) must involve consideration of one critical issue: safety. Controversy concerning eccentric use has concentrated on safety, which supports the present need for continued research on eccentrics as well as education about established clinical and scientific principles.

SPECIFICITY OF MUSCULAR TRAINING

The benefit of mixed mode (muiltimodal) muscle training during rehabilitation has been widely supported,[3–6] and eccentric loading provides one specialized element of a balanced, eclectic rehabilitation or performance program.

In a general sense, the well-established prin-

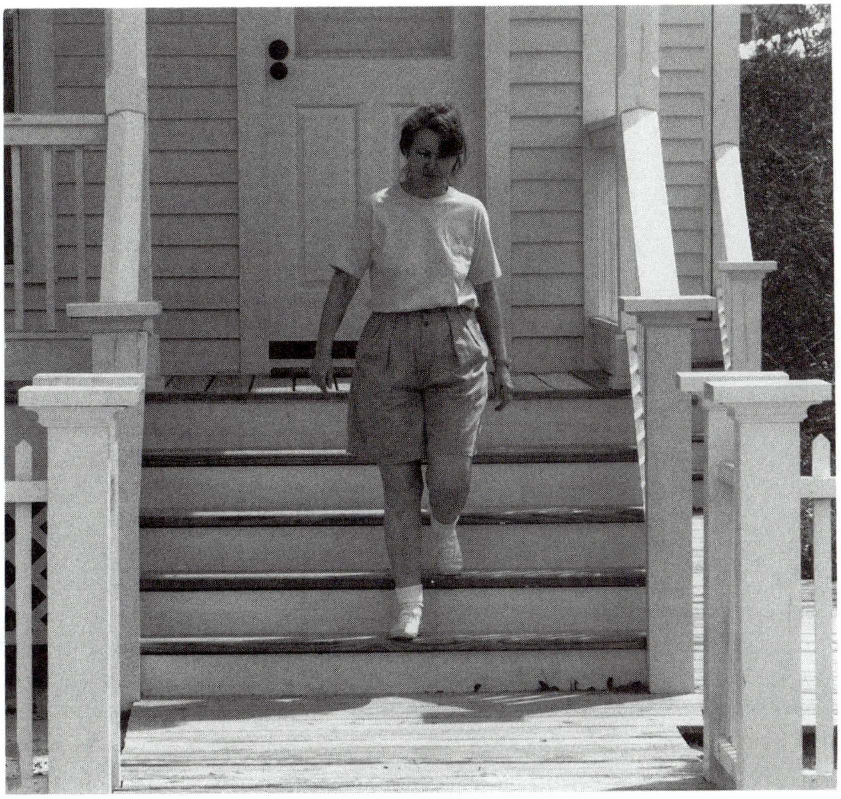

Fig. 1-2. Descending stairs as an example of functional negative work.

Table 1-2. Overview Summary of Resistive Exercise Systems

Isokinetic/Hydraulic	Isotonic Cam Systems (Pulleys, Plates)
Biodex	Dynacam
Cybex[a]	Body Masters
Kin-Com	Adonis
Lido	Paramount
Merac[a]	Polaris
Omnitron	Sprint
Isotechnologies[a]	Nautilus
Biokinetics[a]	Eagle
Ariel[a]	Marcy
Eric[a]	Universal
Isopower[a]	Norsk
Keiser	Isofitness
Bionex[a]	Toro
Hydra-gym	Magnum II

[a] Concentric only.

ciple of specificity[7–10] underlies most decisions about muscular training. The principle of specificity dictates that training modes and testing techniques simulate the functional demands as closely as possible. In addition, the type of muscular contraction, energy system, and neuromuscular control patterns used during training must be replicated by the testing methods to assure valid application of the results to clinical decisions. For instance, the use of eccentric training will optimally prepare the person during moments when an eccentric contraction is required for efficient and safe sports or functional demands. It appears that a functional eccentric contraction is selectively recruited during any activity that involves sudden change in the momentum (the product of the mass of a body and either the linear or angular velocity).[11] This principle applies whether the momentum change is vertical, linear, or rotatory and

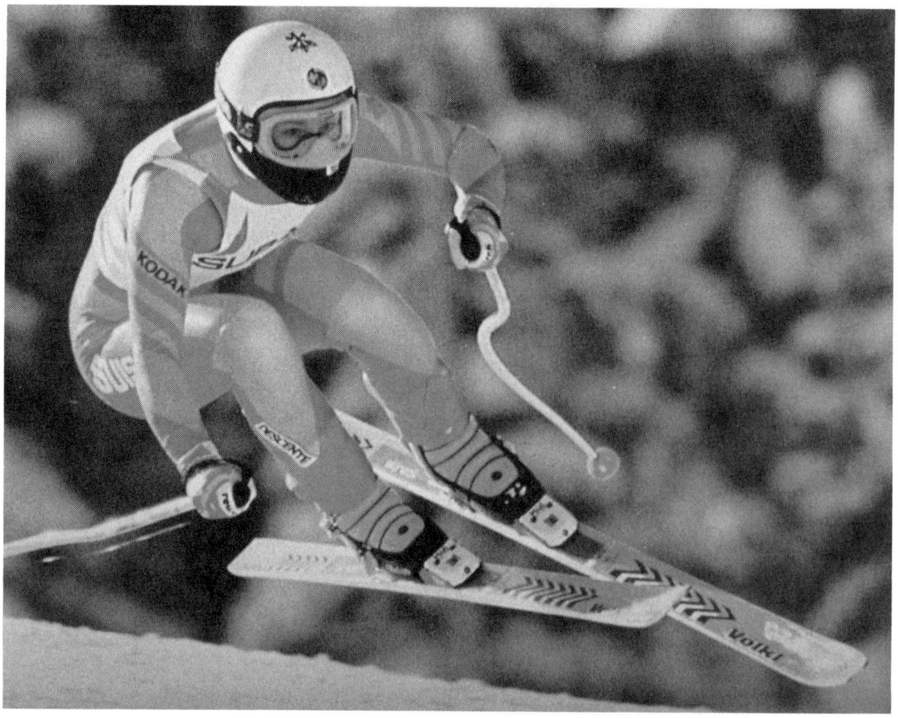

Fig. 1-3. Landing demands.

will affect the human body, limb segment, or various implements involved.

PERSPECTIVES IN THE LITERATURE

Several investigators have discussed the important role of eccentrics in rehabilitation and testing. Dean[12] has encouraged the increased use of eccentrics, while Hinton[13] has promoted eccentric testing to improve understanding of rotator cuff function in the shoulder. Jobe et al.[14] have also described a specific eccentric role in the shoulder during the throwing mechanism. Zarins et al.[15] also review the concept of deceleration from the rotator cuff as an important biomechanical component of overhead throwing motions and other activities that cause many shoulder pathologies.

Multiple studies[16–20] have reported specific eccentric biased principles in the lower extremity, with common references to the patellar tendon. Phillips and Roberts[21] discuss a major role of lower extremity eccentric muscular contraction to control inertia of the leg segment during gait. The complex determinants of muscle action and biomechanics of gait provide an extensive area for research on eccentrics and associated future clinical applications. In addition, the role of eccentric loads in the causation of muscle strains and tears and the importance of specific preventive eccentric training programs have been stressed.[22,23]

The eccentric role in spine function has been sparsely investigated, and support for clinical exercise programs to alter hypermobility or hypomobility or to decrease mechanical strain on injured tissues is lacking. Saudek and Palmer[24] discuss an eccentric function of the multifidi to stabilize the spine during combined flexion and rotation moments, while Troup and Chapman[25] describe a neuromuscular phenomenon in which prime movers about the spine function in eccentric

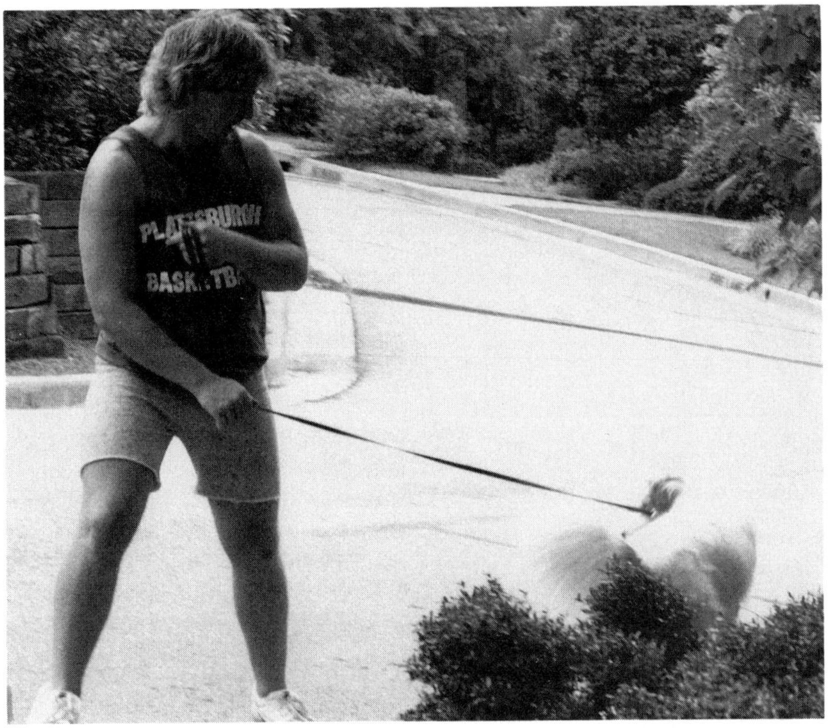

Fig. 1-4. Restraining demands with dog on a leash.

modes during high speed, critical moments in given movement patterns.

With most trunk motions occurring in functional patterns from vertical to 45 degrees of flexion, it is conceivable that lumbar extensors can function eccentrically to lower the trunk. Ashton and Singh[26] identified the lumbar extensors as producing more tension eccentrically than either isometric or concentric contractions, with corresponding low myoelectrical activities.

ECCENTRICS INVOLVEMENT IN TENDONITIS

Clinical and empirical references regarding the important role of eccentric loading in both the etiology and proposed treatment of tendonitis problems are abundant.[15–20,27–30] The histopathology of tendon is dependent on the key capacity of the parallel alignment of its collagen fibers to safely bear tensile loads. Elliot[31] describes the peak capacity of normal tendon as to 48 to 98 newtons per square millimeter. Unfortunately, tendon is poorly vascularized and poorly resistant to the common stresses of compression and shear.

Altered biomechanics due to postural deficits or anatomic deviations, coupled with the loss of muscular protection in cases of disrupted normative agonist to antagonist force ratios, or inappropriate concentric to eccentric force ratios, can clearly produce abnormal shear and compression loads to tendon tissue.

Additionally, as a chief structure of the series elastic component, tendon is selectively stressed during periods of external loading on the body or limb segment from gravity and inertial forces. The role of flexibility becomes important in tendon's capacity to resist injury for two primary reasons. First, the ability of a muscle with a given cross-

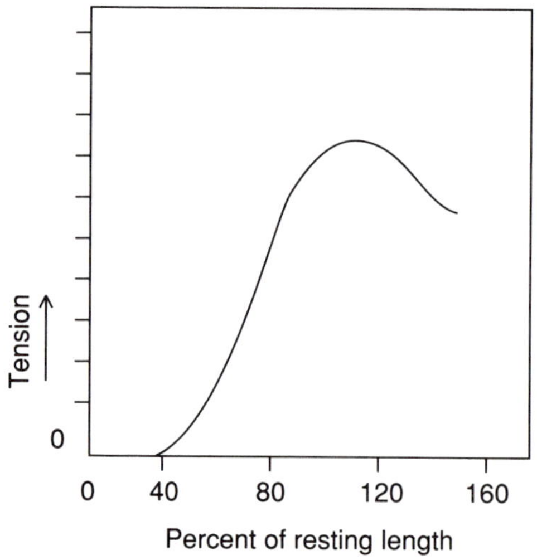

Fig. 1-5. Resting muscle length versus tension. (From Fox et al.,[40] with permission.)

sectional area to create tension is dependent on the muscle achieving optimal length (up to 130 percent of resting length) (Fig. 1-5) immediately prior to contraction. Of course, flexibility deficits can compromise this important prestretch concept. Second, optimal flexibility provides a safety margin for the high tensile forces that result from high-speed reversals of limb motion (eccentric to concentric).

A potentially important predictor and clinical parameter with tendon injury is the "critical deficit" as identified by Bennett and Stauber[27] with respect to anterior knee pain or infrapatellar tendon dysfunctions. The *critical deficit* is a percentage value derived by dividing eccentric force values of a specific muscle or group by the concentric forces of the same muscle. Bennett and Stauber indicated the critical deficit of the knee for eccentric quadriceps torque divided by concentric quadriceps torque to be 85 percent. Although a recent article by Trudelle-Jackson[28] chal-

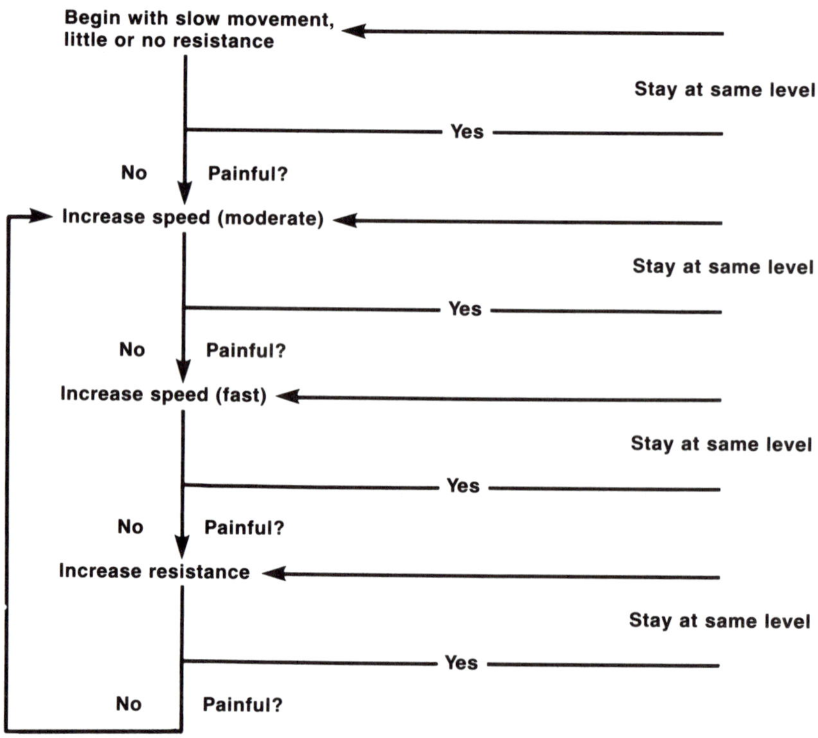

Fig. 1-6. Outline of eccentric exercise program for tendonitis. (From Curwin and Stanish,[29] with permission.)

lenges the accuracy of critical deficit as applied to anterior knee pain, the concept of a predictive relationship between eccentric and concentric force values for a given muscle holds tremendous potential for improving future rehabilitation and training programs. Indeed, the establishment of normative eccentric/concentric force ratios for all skeletal muscles may offer the clinician a powerful new parameter to assist in performance, injury prevention, and rehabilitation settings, and warrants definitive research efforts.

Despite minimal research verification, an excellent clinical approach to tendonitis is offered by Curwin and Stanish.[29] Based on biomechanical and progressive principles, Curwin and Stanish describe a protocol that incorporates the interactive effects of limb speed and resistance loads to progressively train the tensile tolerance of tendon. Resistance loads are selectively biased toward the eccentric mode (Fig. 1-6). I have found this protocol to be consistently effective with tendonitis of multiple anatomic areas in Blazina's stages 1 and 2.[30]

NEUROLOGIC CONTROL CONCEPTS

Motor control issues with eccentric muscle action are poorly understood and provide a potential productive area for future research designs and clinical applications. One basis of support for the theory that eccentric muscle action occurs through a separate neural control system than that for concentric muscle response is the well-established principles of disparate oxygen requirements and myoelectric activity for eccentrics (see Ch. 2). Another mechanism that may implicate a different neural control is the eccentric involvement in series elastic potential energy increases. Two key studies by Hart et al.[32] and Bennett and Stauber[27] have investigated the neural control component using markedly different approaches. Hart et al. used electromyography (EMG) to record force oscillations before and after cooling of the skin of the contracting quadriceps. The consistent finding of decreased force after cooling led the authors to conclude that eccentrics was mediated neurologically. Bennett and Stauber also used quadriceps function to assess the critical deficit described in the previous section; the selective force deficit in eccentrics and the rapid resolution of normal forces after training indicated that the neural system was involved. Laycoe and Marteniuk[33] also attributed training increases with eccentric forces in the quadriceps to neural elements. Moritani et al.[34] examined an upper extremity muscle group, the biceps brachii, and again determined a differential neurologic effect between eccentric and concentric force by EMG assessment. The mechanism of neural control remains unclear and warrants continued experimental research. Several proposed concepts of the mechanism are reviewed in Chapter 2.

SPECIAL CONSIDERATIONS

Recently, the concepts of closed kinetic chain biomechanics and rehabilitation have been popularized in the literature and postgraduate seminars. Closed kinetic activities involve integration of muscle joints acting in sequential order with combined weight bearing and shear forces that are mediated by eccentric muscle action. Although research on the effects of closed chain principles is minimal, apparent clinical success with late stage rehabilitation and functional training (or progressions) indicates the need for continued experimental investigation. Closed chain biomechanics are intricately involved with eccentric muscle control patterns, especially in the lower extremity, and greater attention to the research and clinical application of eccentrics may provide improved protocols for the rehabilitation of many diseases, dysfunctions, and performance skills. The close correlation of closed kinetic chain muscular efficiency with most functional activities of daily living (ADL) and sports demands, and its potential relationship to injury prevention, is an exciting area for progress with therapeutic exercise in the 1990s.

As suggested by Engel[35], chronic diseases often cause debilitating weakness from selective type II muscle fiber atrophy, while Hanid et al.[36] have described similar type II muscle fiber atrophy in alcoholics. Due to the ability to selectively recruit type II fiber, eccentrics may provide a way to ameliorate this weakness.

Yet another important application of eccentric biased training lies in its capacity to effectively modify destructive impulse loads on articular cartilage.[37,38] Hence, the role of eccentric muscle contraction may assist in protection of the joint and prevent eventual dysfunction or even osteoarthritis.[39]

SUMMARY

The role of eccentric muscle loading in multiple functional activities is well supported by the literature, as is the importance of specificity in training. Despite unclear neural control mechanisms, eccentric training affects closed chain biomechanics and tendon function, is an important factor in the management of orthopaedic dysfunctions and injuries and some chronic diseases, and may also act to prevent osteoarthritis. Research and education are needed to further clarify the multiple effects and indications for eccentric biased exercise. The current availability of advanced exercise equipment provides a promising environment for continued investigation and clinical applications.

REFERENCES

1. Stauber WT: Eccentric action of muscles: physiology, injury and adaptation. Exerc Sports Sci Rev 19:157, 1989
2. Rose SJ, Rothstein JR: Muscle biology and physical therapy: A historical perspective. Phys Ther 62:1754, 1982
3. Steadman JR: Rehabilitation of athletic injury. Am J Sports Med 7:147, 1979
4. Costill DL, Fink WJ, Habansky AJ: Muscle rehabilitation after knee surgery. Phys Sports Med 5:71, 1971
5. Hakkinen K, Komi PV: Effect of different combined concentric and eccentric muscle work regimes on maximal strength development. J Human Movement Studies 7:33, 1981
6. Belka D: Comparison of dynamic, static and combination training on dominant wrist flexor muscles. Res Q 39:244, 1968
7. Clarke D, Henry F: Neuro-muscular specificity and increased speed from strength development. Res Q 32:315, 1961
8. Coyle EF, Feiring DC, Cote RW et al: Specificity of power improvements through slow and fast isokinetic movements. J Appl Physiol 51:1437, 1981
9. Gardner G: Specificity of strength changes of the exercised and nonexercised limb following isometric training. Res Q 34:98, 1963
10. Jenkins WL, Thackeberry M, Killian C: Speed-specific isokinetic training. J Orthop Sports Phys Ther 6:181, 1984
11. Enoka RM: Neuro-Mechanical Basis of Kinesiology. Human Kinetics Books, Champaign, IL, 1988
12. Dean E: Physiology and therapeutic implications of negative work. A review. Phys Ther 68:233, 1988
13. Hinton RY: Isokinetic evaluation of shoulder rotational strength in high school baseball pitchers. Am J Sports Med 16:274, 1988
14. Jobe FW, Moynes DR, Tibone JE, Perry J: An EMG analysis of the shoulder in pitching. A second report. Am J Sports Med 12:218, 1984
15. Zarins B, Andrews JR, Carson WG: Injuries to the Throwing Arm. WB Saunders, Philadelphia, 1985
16. Black JE, Alten SR: How I manage infrapatellar tendonitis. Phys Sports Med 12:86, 1984
17. David JM: Jumper's knee. J Orthop Sports Phys Ther 11:137, 1989
18. Hunter SC, Poole RM: The chronically inflamed tendon. Clin Sports Med 6:371, 1987
19. Jensen K, DiFabio RP: Evaluation of eccentric exercises in treatment of patellar tendonitis. Phys Ther 69:211, 1989
20. Stanton P, Purdam C: Hamstring injuries in sprinting—the role of eccentric exercise. J Orthop Sports Phys Ther 10:343, 1989
21. Phillips SJ, Roberts EM, Huang TC: Quantification of intersegmental reactions during rapid swing motion. J Biomech 16:411, 1983
22. Garrett WE: Basic science of musculotendinous injuries. p. 42. In Nicholson JA, Hershman EB (eds): The Lower Extremity and Spine in Sports Medicine. CV Mosby, St. Louis, 1986
23. Duncan PW, Chandler JM, Cavanaugh DK et al.: Mode and speed specificity of eccentric and concentric exercise training. J Orthop Sports Phys Ther 11:70, 1989
24. Saudek CE, Palmer KA: Back pain revisited. J Orthop Sports Phys Ther 8:556, 1987
25. Troup JDG, Chapman AE: The strength of the flexor and extensor muscles of the trunk. J Biomech 2:49, 1969

26. Ashton TEJ, Singh M: Relationship between erectors spinae voltage and backlift strength for isometric, concentric and eccentric contraction. Res Q 46:282, 1975
27. Bennett JG, Stauber WT: Evaluation and treatment of anterior knee pain using eccentric exercise. Med Sci Sports Exerc 18:528, 1986
28. Trudelle-Jackson E, Meske N, Highenboten C et al.: Eccentric-Concentric torque deficits in the quadriceps muscle. J Orthop Sports Phys Ther 11:142, 1989
29. Curwin S, Stanish WD: Tendonitis: Its Etiology and Treatment. DC Heath and Co., Lexington, 1985
30. Blazina ME, Kerlan RK, Jobe FW et al.: Jumper's knee. Orthop Clin North Am 4:665, 1973
31. Elliot DH: Structure and function of mammalian tendon. Biol Rev 40:392, 1965
32. Hart DL, Miller LC, Stauber WT: Effect of cooling on force oscillations during maximal voluntary eccentric exercise. Exp Neurol 90:73, 1985
33. Laycoe RR, Marteniuk RG: Learning and tension as factors in static strength gains produced by static and eccentric training. Res Q 42:299, 1971
34. Moritani T, Muramatsu S, Muro M: Activity of motor units during concentric and eccentric contractions. Am J Phys Med 66:338, 1987
35. Engel WK: Selective and nonselective susceptibility of muscle fiber types. Arch Neurol 22:97, 1970
36. Hanid A, Slavin G, Main W et al.: Fibre type changes in striated muscle of alcoholics. J Clin Pathol 34:991, 1981
37. Radin EL: Aetiology of osteoarthritis. Clin Rheum Dis 3:509, 1976
38. Sirca A, Susec-Michieli M: Selective type II fibre muscular atrophy in patients with osteoarthritis of the hip. J Neurol Sci 301:3, 1977
39. White AA III, Gordon SL: Synopsis: workshop on idiopathic low-back pain. Spine 7:141, 1982
40. Fox EL, Bowers RW, Foss ML: Physiological Basis of Physical Education and Athletics. 4th Ed. WB Saunders, Philadelphia, 1988

2

Physiologic and Clinical Principles of Eccentrics

Since 1953,[1] concepts of the differences between the subtypes of isotonic exercise have been widely investigated in the scientific literature. However, specific use of eccentric biased exercise in the clinical setting was uncommon until the early to mid-1980s.[2] Consequently, the purposes of this chapter are as follows:

1. To compare and contrast concentric with eccentric muscle loading
2. To describe potential advantages and benefits of eccentric exercise
3. To describe principles of eccentric clinical protocols
4. To develop a profile of the mechanical, metabolic, and physiologic parameters of eccentrics

Eccentric muscle activity is most appropriately termed *muscle response,* due to the muscle lengthening during tension production. The unique and differential effects of eccentrics involve a circular interaction of three primary determinants: muscular force, speed of movement, and degree of musculotendinous stretch (Fig. 2-1).

Several interdependent biomechanical determinants provide the basis for the confirmed differences of eccentrics on the human muscular and neuromotor systems. First, there is the *electromechanical delay,*[3] which refers to the elapsed time from biochemical response to actual onset of muscular tension. This delay is shortest for the eccentric mode of contraction, which provides a potential training benefit (see the section *Neuromuscular Control Concepts*). According to Cavanagh and Komi[3] in their study on elbow flexors and extensors, the eccentric mode acted 4.4 milliseconds faster than the isometric mode and 6 milliseconds faster than the concentric contraction, which was statistically significant for both differences.

Second, the *stretch shorten cycle* described by Cavagna et al.[4] is relevant to effects of eccentrics due to its potential for storage and use of elastic energy. In this cycle, the primary volitional movement is preceded by the opposite or antagonistic movement in a rapid manner producing a subsequently greater magnitude of contractile force due to the addition of potential energy transferred from the series elastic component (SEC).[5] This potentiation effect is frequently used in functional activities when prestretch is applied to a given

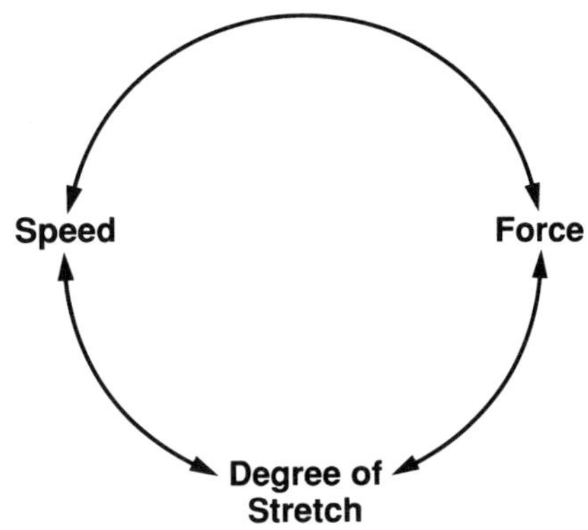

Fig. 2-1. Triumvirate of interactive eccentrics effects.

musculotendinous unit by eccentric response and followed immediately by the counter-concentric contraction. So, briefly stated, the eccentric contraction potentiates the force of the following concentric contraction. For this effect to occur, the conditions of rapid stretch, rapid reversal of movement from eccentric to concentric action, and a short range of movement must exist.[6,7]

The third major principle underlying much of the physiologic differences of eccentric contractions is called the *Elftman proposal*.[8] This principle states that the optimal force production of different modes of contraction is arranged in a predictable hierarchy as follows:

Eccentric → Isometric → Concentric

This predictable relationship has been repeatedly verified by multiple studies[9–17] and appears consistent for all upper extremity, lower extremity, and trunk skeletal muscles. A useful guideline for clinical and training applications states that the peak eccentric force (tension) for any given muscle is 1.8 times the isometric force of the same muscle.[18] The scientific literature regarding eccentrics often interchanges the terms *strength* (or *power*) and *force*. A consensus comparison of force (or, more accurately, the tension capacities of eccentrics with concentrics) is reviewed in Table 2-1.[1,9–17]

Because concentric muscle activity has a maximum achievable tension level, activities that require tension loads exceeding the peak level are met with two compensatory mechanisms. First, additional tension is gained from the summation of momentum from adjacent limb segments in a sequenced manner. Second, additional tension is developed through the addition of potential energy to the SEC (noncontractile elements). A conceptual schematic is presented in Figure 2-2.

The final biomechanical variable for eccentrics involves the efficiency of the crossbridge mechanism in creating force during contraction. During eccentric contraction, it is postulated[19,20] that the crossbridge movement and coupling are able to act at a faster rate, causing a resultant decreased energy requirement from the oxygen system. Adaptations of eccentric muscle action produce an optimal overlay between the actin and myosin elements,[2] which in turn increases peak force potential.

The peculiar high tension of eccentrics relates to the manner in which the crossbridge connections are made and maintained.[21] The economy associated with eccentrics is in part due to the development of tension without the normal re-

Table 2-1. Comparative Eccentric Versus Concentric Force Levels

Reference	Muscle	Force % Eccentric/ Concentric	Speed (degrees per second)	Mode
Denuccio et al.[11]	Quadriceps	187	180	IK
Doss and Karpovich[12]	Elbow flexors	139		IT
Komi and Rusko[13]	Elbow flexors	200	120	IK
Asmussen[1]	Elbow flexors	163		IT
Minor and Soderberg[14]	Ankle plantar flexors	178	12	IK
Griffin[9]	Elbow flexors	112 130 132	30 120 210	IK
Rodgers and Berger[15]	Elbow flexors	200	45	
Gray and Chandler[16]	Quadriceps	146	180	IK
Olson et al.[17]	Hip abduction	162	Not specified	IT
Seliger et al.[10]	Quadriceps	300	17	IK

Abbreviations: IK, isokinetic; IT, isotonic.

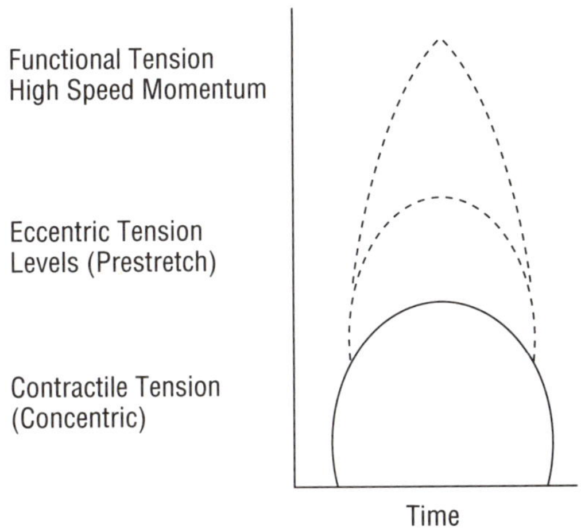

Fig. 2-2. Summation of elastic energy and force.

quirement of splitting adenosine triphosphate (ATP) or creatine phosphate (CP).[22]

PHYSIOLOGIC PRINCIPLES

This section reviews and highlights the significant areas of physiologic, biomechanical, and clinical characteristics of eccentric muscle loading. Efficiency of muscular action[15,23–26] is a primary feature of eccentrics and is explained by many interrelated effects. Clinical applications of eccentric loading are strongly supported by this inherent efficiency.

Electromyogram Considerations

Asmussen[1] reported higher electromyogram (EMG) activity for concentric work of a given resistance load than for eccentrics, which is consistently supported by other studies.[10,27] Studies by Bigland and Lippold[28] and Matsui et al.[29] found that the EMG activity for concentrics exceeded that for eccentrics by a two- to threefold factor. More recent studies[30,31] have demonstrated similar EMG activity for eccentric and isometric responses, with the highest activity also found for concentrics (Fig. 2-3). Komi and Viitasalo[32] found that the EMG measurements after eccentric work demonstrated weakened response, or fatigue, of the neuromuscular system for 2 days after the work bout.

One interesting variation between eccentrics and concentrics was a progressive increase of integrated EMG during continued eccentric exercise with no significant increase in the concentric condition.[28] Komi and Rusko,[13] however, found equal decreases in integrated EMG activity after 4 repeat bouts of 40 repetitions with the biceps.

Finally, the level of EMG activity with a given muscular response appears more dependent on the subjects degree of effort than on the amount of tension generated.[30]

Oxygen Utilization

Knuttgen et al.[33] determined that comparable work values required 70 to 75 percent less oxygen for eccentrics than for concentrics (Fig. 2-4), Knuttgen et al. also stated that eccentrics performed to exhaustion relative to oxygen supply could readily produce tissue damage or orthopaedic problems. Davies and Barnes[34] reported that eccentric exercise for downhill walking required only 20 percent of the oxygen consumption compared with concentrics at the same intensity levels.

A separate perspective describes the oxygen uptake per unit of muscle activity to be three times greater for concentric activity.[35] The oxygen uptake per unit of muscular activity has been consistently shown to be decreased as a result of training with eccentrics.[36,37] Davies and Barnes concluded that the training effects were caused by muscular system adaptations and were not the result of circulatory or respiratory changes. An important consideration for oxygen uptake during any type of peripheral joint muscular work involves the corresponding work of the spinal and hip musculature in isometric, stabilizing functions.

During exhaustive, prolonged eccentric work bouts the cardiac frequency (pulse rate) was near maximum, while the subject was performing at only 60 percent of his maximum aerobic power.[36] Bonde-Peterson et al.[37] determined that during

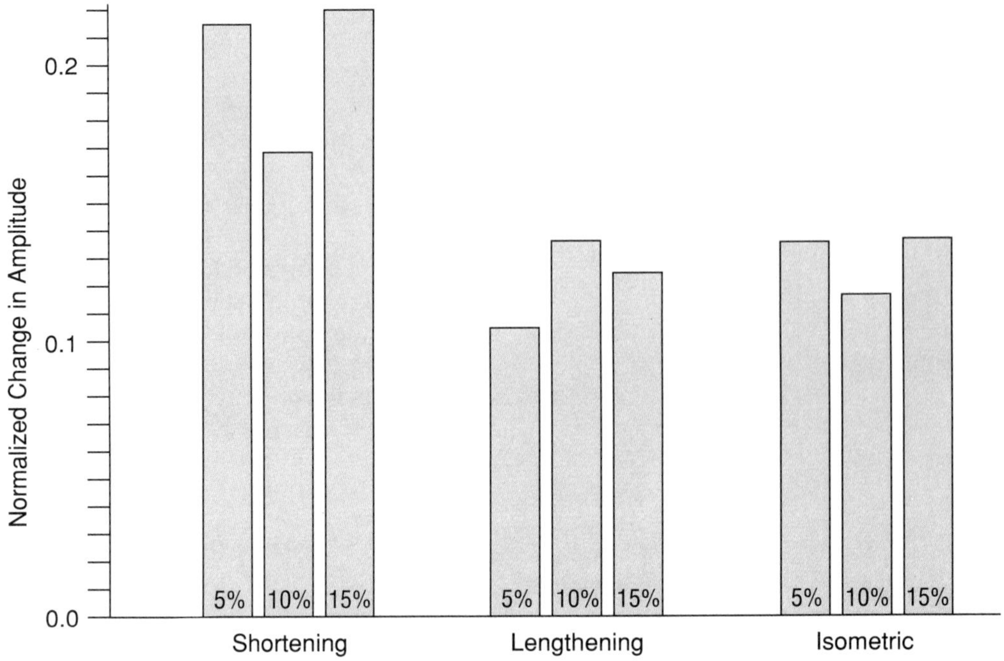

Fig. 2-3. EMG activity with three different muscle loads. (From Andrew,[30] with permission.)

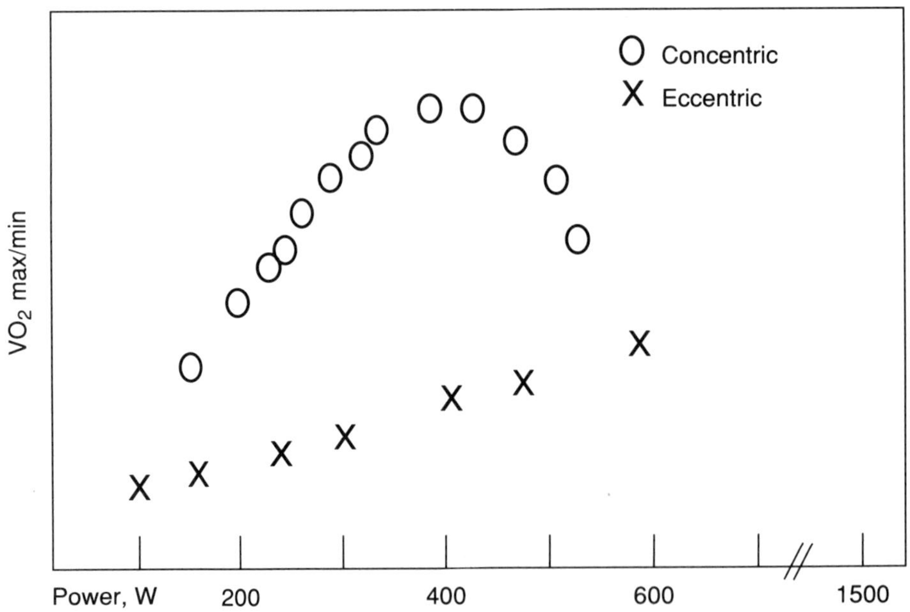

Fig. 2-4. Oxygen uptake at various force levels. (From Knuttgen et al.,[33] with permission.)

steady state oxygen uptake for a 4-minute work bout, high intensity eccentric work was nearly equivalent to low intensity concentric work. Finally, it is apparent that eccentric training is not limited by respiratory or circulatory factors and eccentrics does not produce pronounced training effects on the cardiorespiratory system.

Blood Pressure Effects

Pimental et al.[38] found that eccentrics produced a pressor response that would increase mean arterial pressure and heart rate. MacDougall et al.[39] described pronounced hemodynamic changes with the use of free weight lifts (with an eccentric phase) in experienced subjects; such use caused blood pressure elevations to 320/250 mmHg due to a combination of the pressor effect and the Valsalva effect. A rapid decline of these elevated pressures occurred during the eccentric phase, which suggests that blood pressure is more dependent on effort than the amount of muscular tension.

These documented hemodynamic alterations from eccentric exercise support the importance of correct rhythmic breathing mechanics during exercise. The eccentric phase of an exercise should be preceded by a deep inspiration that produces a strong stabilizing "tightness" (D. Pasanella, personal communication, Atlanta, 1990). The subsequent push phase or concentric movement is supplemented by a strong exhalation, or "push" breath. Appropriate breathing becomes paramount in patients who are deconditioned, elderly, or have high blood pressure, and in people who are unaccustomed to resistive exercise training.

Body Temperature Changes and Adjustments

Body temperature regulation is a complex balance between central and peripheral influences according the principles of Benzinger.[40] The relative absence of lactate concentration in the blood in eccentrics demonstrates that blood flow is adequate during exhaustive exercise. Since mechanical influences during eccentric exercise actually cause work to be done on the muscle, as opposed to by the muscle, this transfer of energy is responsible for an increase in body temperature. Nielsen et al.[41] demonstrated a threefold greater heat production for an equal level of eccentric exercise. The increase in body heat requires that heat be eliminated from the skin, which has an adequate compensatory blood supply, producing the characteristic early and extensive sweat production. Internal or core temperature during eccentric exercise remained lower than during concentrics,[42] perhaps due to the lower muscle blood requirements. At any body temperature, the skin temperature during eccentric work exceeded that experienced during concentric work by 3 degrees centigrade, and the muscle temperature was 1.2 degrees centigrade higher for eccentrics than for concentrics.[43] In addition, the increase in muscle temperature during the transient phase of initial exercise was more rapid for eccentric loads. Pahud et al.[44] verified the accuracy of an energy balance equation that specifies that during eccentric work the mechanical energy absorbed by the body tissues must be stored or dissipated as heat (Fig. 2-5).

Psychological Parameters and Significance

A key concept in the use of eccentric biased exercise is the effects of this type of muscle action on the subject's rating of perceived exertion (RPE). The eventual outcome of physical training programs is dependent on subject compliance with continued exercise and motivational levels that are sufficient for intense efforts. Eccentric muscle loading possesses several characteristics of pyschological perception and tolerance. Mannheimer[45] claimed that subjects felt they might be "overcome" by a load in the lowering action and felt they had to fight off the weight in a self-protective mechanism. A protective reaction could be seen to produce a higher level of effort and perhaps arousal from fear of injury, which in turn could cause a training overload stimulus. Some individuals perceive a stretching force that is fast or that exceeds 140 percent of their 1-repetition maximum concentric force as being un-

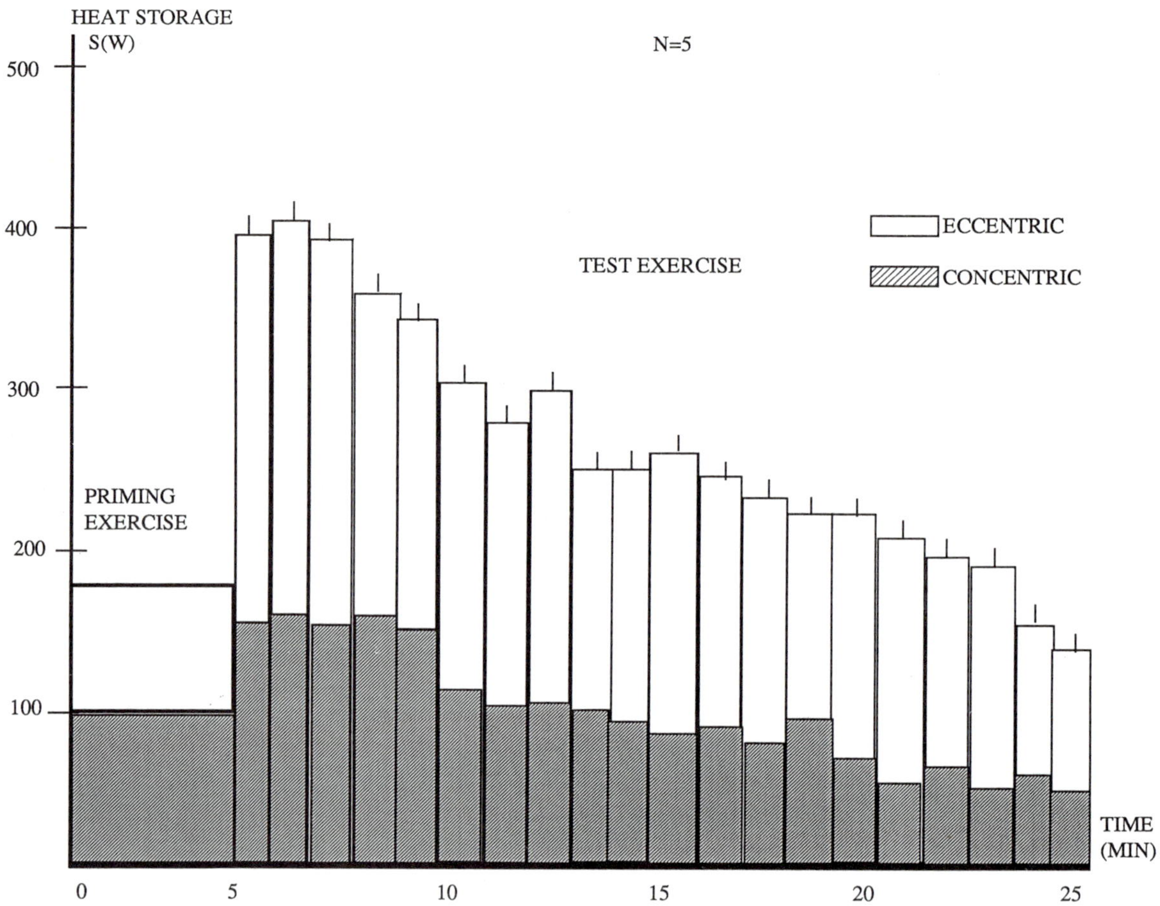

Fig. 2-5. Heat production with eccentric muscle loading. (From Pahud et al.,[44] with permission.)

controlled and, therefore, inhibitory.[46,47] Johnson[48] stated that eccentric muscle loads felt easier to perform than concentrics, while Newham et al.[49] described eccentrics as feeling effortless. Newham et al.[50] also reported feelings of weakness and instability in the working muscle after repetitive stepping exercises. This feeling corresponds to a shaky sensation, or "rubber legs."

By contrast, Eloranta and Komi[51] and Hendrickson et al.[52] stated that eccentrics was perceived as greater exertion when compared with concentrics as related to heart rate and oxygen uptake. A possible explanation for a heightened perception of exertion may be caused by peripheral impulses from increased mechanoreceptor stimuli in the SEC.[21]

Training with eccentrics produces a decrease in the perceived exertion for the same intensity load.[53] Clinical observation shows that initial training with only an eccentric pattern feels unnatural to the subject and produces a shaky muscular response that is uncoordinated and may be accompanied by subject distress. With verbal assurance, most subjects will become psychologically confident and display increased control within 3 to 5 repetitions. Based on these observations, it is wise to precede maximal or heavy eccentric training with several submaximal trials, both for neuromotor cueing and small temperature increases that can facilitate visco-elastic properties.

Another important consideration in regard to the pyschological effects of eccentric training involves the higher intrinsic tension that can be produced. In the case of the low-motivated subject (one who finds resistive exercise difficult because of disinterest, secondary gain from disability, weakness, pain with specific movements, or altered arthrokinematics), eccentrics may provide an immediate success by controlling a weight that could not be mastered concentrically. This successful completion of a new resistive task can start a positive feedback or reinforcement loop, which in turn leads to increased strength and motivation and overall program compliance. Improved patient mood and affect are attributed to increased functional status and independence, thus creating a self-perpetuating cycle.[26]

Human perception of exertion levels arise from an integration of impulses from pain and thermal receptors, mechanoreceptors, baroreceptors, chemoreceptors, and the brain. Consequently, Andrew's[30] finding of a marked variation between RPE for eccentric and concentric loading is understandable.

Muscular Endurance Factors

Komi and Viitasalo[32] found slow velocity isokinetic eccentric contractions to be highly fatiguing due to the high degree of SEC tension. Gray and Chandler[16] found that high speed eccentric contractions were more fatigue resistant than the concentric fatigue rate for quadriceps. The greater fatigue found during slow velocity eccentrics may be explained by the lack of optimal force potentiation associated with high speed reversal of the stretch-shorten cycle.[32] Eccentric muscle loading requires lower energy utilization (ATP and CP), which supports delayed fatigue responses in anaerobically contracting muscle.

Newham et al.[50] described the differential behavior of eccentrically fatigued muscle in terms of response to electrical stimulation. Eccentrically fatigued muscle showed dramatic decreases in force during low frequency (10 Hz) stimulation but not during high frequency (50 Hz) stimulation. This differential fatigue response was most pronounced at 1 hour postexercise and normalized at 24 hours, as with concentrics. Newham et al. also described decreases in maximal voluntary force that were statistically significant only in the eccentrically fatigued muscles and again, they normalized within 24 hours. One explanation for this finding involves mechanical damage to the sarcoplasmic reticulum with altered calcium release and corresponding nerve electrical activity.[2]

Perhaps the use of low frequency electrical stimulation may be effective in treating posteccentric exercise soreness. Future research on this topic should investigate various electrical wave parameters and types of electrical mode (i.e., high volt galvanic, low volt).

Velocity Attributes

As early as 1952, Abbott et al.[54] described the inverse relationship of force versus velocity between concentric and eccentric muscular responses, with a finite limit to the degree to which eccentric force rises at higher speeds. Currently, the eccentric force-velocity curve is a controversial issue, with the primary question being whether there is a limit or plateau to eccentric forces, or a continued exponential increase in force with a higher speed of movement. Key considerations of the force-velocity relationship for eccentrics include whether the contraction mode is isotonic or isokinetic, and the speed of motion used.

Using isotonic modes, Asmussen et al.,[55] Komi,[25] and Komi and Buskirk[56] reported increased eccentric force with increased velocity of movement. Eloranta and Komi[51] and Jorgensen[57] reported highest forces at slow velocities with reductions (statistically nonsignificant) in force at higher speeds. Two isokinetic studies[56,58] demonstrated increased force as speed increased, while Hageman et al.[59] found no significant changes or lower extremity torque from 30 to 180 degrees per second. It should be noted that the studies[56,58] that found a direct relationship between force and speed of movement used extremely slow speeds (on the order of 30 degrees per second and slower), which may influence the generalization of results to clinical practice concerns.

Despite the limited research in this specific area of eccentric behavior, there are mixed and conflicting results that fuel controversy over clinical applications. The literature discusses varied test positions, different testing instruments and body positions, different muscle groups, and widely varied speeds and contraction modes. Continued research using clinical approaches is needed and will provide new direction for clinical guidelines in eccentric program design. Improved scientific background on questions of specific eccentric force-velocity characteristics of muscles and of training effects on physiologic overflow across speeds would clarify clinical rationale and maximize the effectiveness of training for both optimal time and safety considerations (see Ch. 3).

Neuromuscular Control Concepts

For purposes of clarification, the terms *neuromuscular* and *neuromotor* will be used in a synonomous and interchangeable manner. Of all the physiologic effects of eccentrics reviewed in this chapter, it is clear that the neuromuscular characteristics of eccentric muscle loading are the least understood.[32] Unfortunately, neuromotor mechanisms have great significance in the understanding of training effects with eccentrics and, indeed, may serve to explain the scientifically verified differences as described in the previous sections.

Key concepts that influence the mechanisms of eccentric neuromuscular control center around three separate, but perhaps interdependent, factors:

1. Altered mechanoreceptor activity (i.e., tendon reflexes)[60]
2. Changes in myoelectric and neural activity and muscle recruitment
3. Altered viscoelastic responses

Whether eccentric neural changes are central[21] or peripheral[32] is an issue that is presently undecided. Hart et al.[60] investigated cooling effects of the skin and concluded that eccentric force oscillations were decreased and EMG responses were altered. Changes in the sensitivity of muscle spindles were associated with the observed results. In addition, both Bonde-Peterson et al.[53] and Stauber[2] concluded that neuromotor changes occurred on a peripheral basis.

Knuttgen and Klausen[21] implicated a unique efferent control mechanism in eccentrics caused by the increased mechanoreceptor input associated with the three- to fivefold greater muscle fiber tension levels when compared with concentrics. The increased mechanoreceptor activity was postulated to be from the Golgi tendon organ (GTO), which would alter the muscular recruitment patterns.

In eccentrics, the central nervous system (CNS) possesses a protective mechanism during peak loads that prevent complete rupture of muscles. Therefore, the force-velocity relationship would not produce an exponentially increased force during increased speeds, but would demonstrate a plateau followed by a sudden loss of force. This "clasped knife reflex"[61] is analogous to the feel of a sudden "soft" loss of resistance experienced when closing a pocket knife. The clasp knife reflex operates as an override circuit (GTO inhibitory mechanism) that occurs only after substantial muscle stretch has occurred.[2] This inherent threshold effect of "safe" stretch provides functional efficiency and is a chief byproduct of eccentric training.

Muscle spindle activity may govern the rate of passive stretch of the SEC through the efficient storage and utilization of potential energy.[62] Muscle spindles seem restricted to slow twitch areas of muscles,[62] while slow acting muscles (i.e., the deltoid) have high spindle indexes.[63] This may indicate that fast twitch fiber or fast acting muscle is dependent to a greater extent on the GTO for neuromuscular control.

Many investigators suggest the preferential recruitment of fast twitch or type II muscle fibers with eccentric muscle loading.[6,64,65] Consistent with fast twitch recruitment are the observations that eccentrics produce greater force throughout a given range of motion[66] and lower work or average torque levels,[16] corresponding to a "spiky" appearance of the force curve shape (Fig. 2-6). Stauber[2] recognized the rapid recruitment of additional muscle fibers at submaximal EMG levels as a correlate of the muscular damage resulting

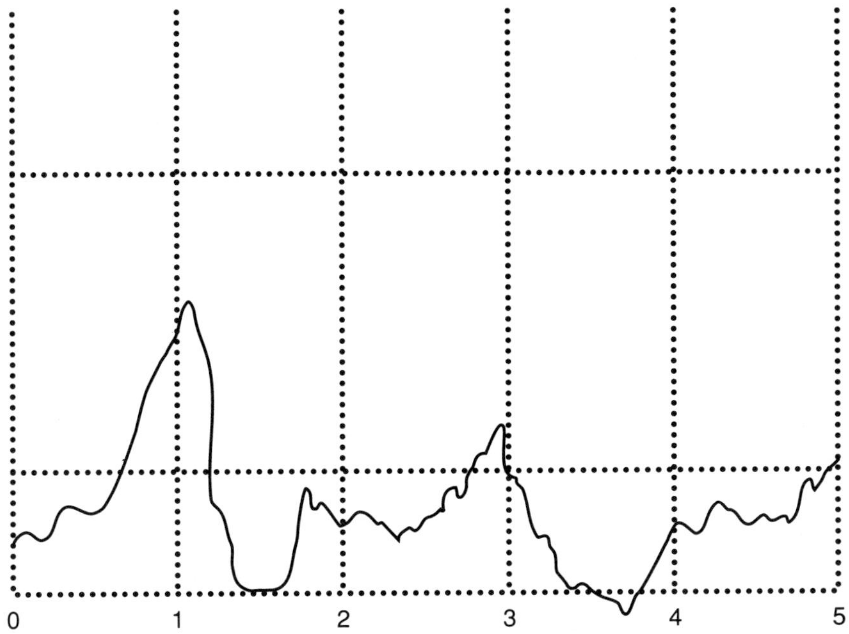

Fig. 2-6. Force curve for eccentric response (classic "spiky" shape).

from eccentric training. The role of recruitment of additional fibers as opposed to rate modulation in order to achieve increased submaximal force is considered controversial and unverified.[30]

An important role of eccentric training on the neuromuscular system is supported by Bennett and Stauber[66] through two mechanisms:

1. Suppression of torque was evident only during eccentric loads, regardless of biomechanical dysfunction or pain.
2. Successful response to eccentric training in only 2 to 4 weeks corresponds to the time frame for neuromuscular adaptation as opposed to a hypertrophy or morphologic change.[67]

As the final factor in neuromuscular control, viscoelasticity may be altered by changes in the threshold level of the GTO[6,54] Viscoelastic stiffness, defined as the resultant level of muscular tension per unit of imposed stretch, is increased during eccentric muscular responses. Crossbridge formation will increase the stiffness of muscle, while elongation will tend to increase the tension of a strongly activated muscle.[68]

Norman and Komi[62] described the speed of muscle stretch as the key determinant in electromechanical delay (EMD). Increasing the velocity with biceps eccentrics caused the EMD to decrease from 38 to 28 milliseconds. Interestingly, the triceps, although classified as a more fast twitch predominate muscle than the biceps by Johnson et al.,[69] demonstrated a similiar EMD time of 30 milliseconds. The possibility that fast speed eccentrics can modify the characteristic velocity attributes of particular muscles deserves further research due to significant potential for clinical and functional training benefits. In addition, Cummings (personal communication, Atlanta, 1990) describes the behavior of collagen as possibly being the limiting factor in force development.

Summary

For purposes of comparison, the scientific literature regarding eccentrics can be categorized into either a classical (the mid-1950s to 1975) or a neo-

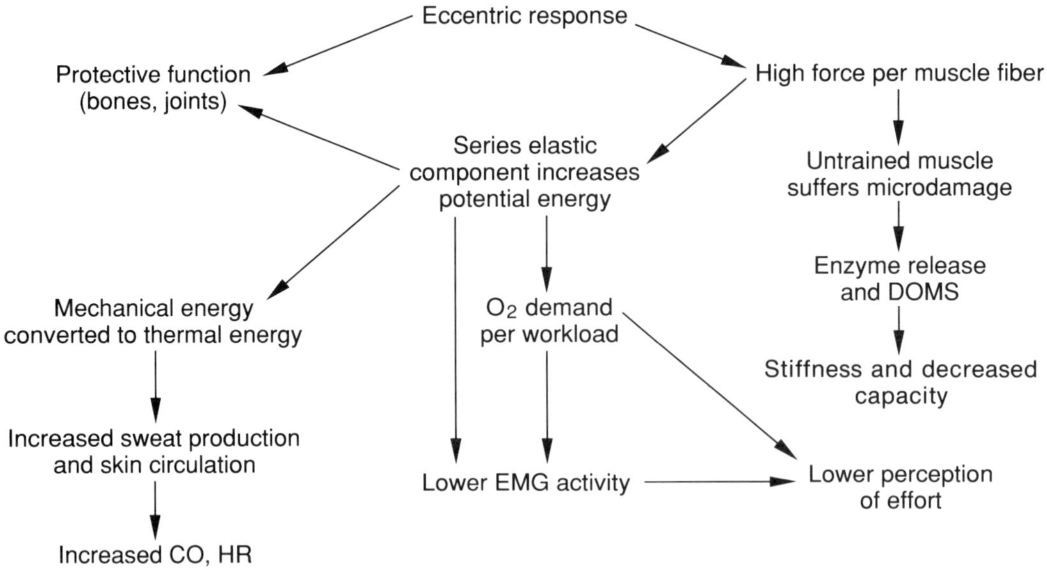

Fig. 2-7. Flow chart of eccentric responses.

classical period (1975 to the present). These periods represent the evolution of the understanding of eccentrics, including current clinical applications. The classical period involved works (led by the prolific works of Paavo Komi) that centered on multiple organ system responses to eccentric loading that were usually of slow speed, repetitive, and sustained in nature. Many of these studies used functional methods or specially made dynamometers and ergometers. Despite the establishment of many important principles, these studies also led to the initial awareness of the muscular damage associated with eccentrics and the resultant delayed onset muscle soreness (DOMS) (see Ch. 3). This concept may have forestalled clinical usage due to perceived risk.

In contrast, the neoclassical period concentrated on the effects and responses of eccentrics on the musculotendinous unit with varied studies on torque, speed, and joint angles through use of objective, reliable isokinetic dynamometers, such as the Kin-Com (see Ch. 6). Due to numerous methodologic differences, these muscular force studies produced controversial results on some issues, but also provided initial guidelines for effective clinical use.

While neuromuscular control of eccentrics is poorly understood, the three primary areas of mechanisms (viscoelastic changes, mechanoreceptor effects, and myoelectric/recruitment alterations) provide the basis for research on the training adaptations from eccentrics as well as the events of DOMS (see Ch. 3).

A schematic flow chart is presented as an overview of the multiple, interactive physiologic effects and responses of eccentric muscle loading (Fig. 2-7).

REFERENCES

1. Asmussen E: Positive and negative work. Acta Physiol Scand 28:364, 1953
2. Stauber WT: Eccentric action of muscles: physiology, injury and adaptation. Exerc Sports Sci Rev 19:157, 1989
3. Cavanagh PR, Komi PV: Electro-chemical delay in human skeletal muscle under concentric and eccentric contractions. Eur J Appl Physiol 42:159, 1979
4. Cavagna GA, Saibene FP, Margaria R: Effect of negative work on the amount of positive work performed by an isolated muscle. J Appl Physiol 20:157, 1965
5. Asmussen E, Bonde-Peterson F: Storage of elastic

energy in skeletal muscles in man. Acta Physiol 91:385, 1974
6. Bosco C, Komi PV, Ito A: A prestretch potentiation of human skeletal muscle during ballistic movement. Acta Physiol Scand 111:135, 1981
7. Bosco C, Viitasalo JT, Komi PV, Luhtanen P: Combined effect of elastic energy and myoelectrical potentiation during stretch shortening cycle exercise. Acta Physiol Scand 114:557, 1982
8. Elftman H: Biomechanics of muscle. J Bone Joint Surg 48:363, 1966
9. Griffin JW: Differences in elbow flexion torque measured concentrically, eccentrically and isometrically. Phys Ther 67:1205, 1987
10. Seliger V, Dolejs L, Karas V: A dynamometric comparison of maximum eccentric, concentric and isometric contractions using emg and energy expenditure measurements. Eur J Appl Physiol 45:235, 1980
11. DeNuccio DK, Davies GJ, Rowinski MJ: Comparison of quadriceps isokinetic concentric contraction data using a standard fatigue protocol. Phys Ther 66:794, 1986
12. Doss WS, Karpovich PV: A comparison of concentric, eccentric and isometric strength of elbow flexors. J Appl Physiol 20:351, 1965
13. Komi PV, Rusko H: Quantitative evaluation of mechanical and electrical changes during fatigue loading of eccentric and work. Scand J Rehabil Med, suppl. 3:S121, 1974
14. Minor SD, Soderberg GL: Isokinetic concentric and eccentric forces in ankle plantarflexion. Phys Ther 67:753, 1987
15. Rodgers KL, Berger RA: Motor unit involvement and tension during maximum voluntary concentric, eccentic and isometric contraction of the elbow flexors. Med Sci Sports Exerc 6:253, 1974
16. Gray JC, Chandler JM: Percent decline in peak torque production during repeated concentric and eccentric contractions of the quadricep femoris muscle. J Orthop Sports Phys Ther 10:309, 1989
17. Olson VL, Smidt GL, Johnston R: The maximum torque generated by the eccentric, isometric and concentric contractions of the hip abductor muscles. Phys Ther 52:149, 1972
18. Abbott BC, Aubert XM, Hill AV: The absorption of work by a muscle stretched during a single twitch or a short tetanus. Proc R Soc B 139:86, 1951
19. Flitney FW, Hirst DG: Tension responses and sarcomere movements during length changes applied to contracting frog's muscle. J Physiol (Lond) 251:66, 1975
20. Joyce GC, Rack PMH, Westbury DR: The mechanical properties of cat soleus muscle during controlled lengthening and shortening movements. J Physiol 204:461, 1969
21. Knuttgen HG, Klausen K: Oxygen debt in short-term exercise with concentric and eccentric muscle contractions. J Appl Physiol 30:632, 1971
22. Curtin NA, Svensson SMM, Davies RE: Force development and the braking mechanism in stretching is not limited by the energy from atp splitting, abstracted. Fed Proc 29:714, 1970
23. Knuttgen HG, Petersen FB, Klausen K: Exercise with concentric and eccentric muscle contractions. Acta Paediatr Scand, suppl. 42:S217, 1971
24. Kaneko M, Komi PV, Aura O: Mechanical efficiency of concentric and eccentric exercises performed with medium to fast contraction rates. Scand J Sports Sci 6:15, 1984
25. Komi PV: Measurement of the force-velocity relationship in human muscle under concentric and eccentric contractions. Med Sports:Biomechanics III 8:224, 1973
26. Dean E: Physiology and therapeutic implications of negative work. Phys Ther 68:233, 1988
27. Basmajian JV: Muscles Alive. Their Functions Revealed by Electromyography. 2nd Ed. Williams & Wilkins, Baltimore, 1967
28. Bigland B, Lippold OCJ: The relation between force, velocity and integrated electrical activity in human muscles. J Physiol 123:214, 1954
29. Matsui H, Miyashita M, Mochinoshi M, Hoskikava T: The electromyographic study of positive and negative work, p. 36. In: Copies of our Researches. University Press, Nagoya, 1970
30. Andrew PD: Motor unit activity under low tensions as muscle changes length. Am J Phys Med 64:235, 1985
31. Heckathorne CW, Childress DS: Relationships of the surface electro-myogram to force, length, velocity and contaction rate of the cineplastic human biceps. Am J Phys Med 60:1, 1981
32. Komi PV, Viitasalo JT: Changes in motor unit activity and metabolism in human skeletal muscle during and after repeated eccentric and concentric contractions. Acta Physiol Scand 100:246, 1977
33. Knuttgen HG, Patton JF, Vogel JA: An ergometer for concentric and eccentric muscular exercise. J Appl Physiol 53:784, 1982
34. Davies CTM, Barnes C: Negative (eccentric) work. Physiological responses to walking uphill and downhill on a motordriven treadmill. Ergonomics 15:121, 1972

35. Bigland-Ritchie B, Woods JJ: Integrated electromyogram and oxygen uptake during positive and negative work. J Physiol 260:267, 1976
36. Davies CTM, Barnes C: Negative (eccentric) work. I. Effects of repeated exercise. Ergonomics 15:3, 1972
37. Bonde-Peterson F, Knuttgen HG, Hendriksson J: Muscle metabolism during exercise with concentric and eccentric contractions. J Appl Physiol 33:792, 1972
38. Pimental NA, Shapiro Y, Pandolf KB: Comparison of uphill and downhill walking and concentric and eccentic cycling. Ergonomics 25:373, 1982
39. MacDougall JD, Tuxen D, Sale DG et al: Arterial blood pressure responses to heavy resistance exercise. J Appl Physiol 58:785, 1985
40. Benzinger TH: The thermostatic regulation of human heat production and heat loss. Proceedings of the 22nd International Physiological Congress, Leiden. 1:415, 1962
41. Nielsen B, Nielsen SL, Bonde-Peterson F: Thermoregulation during positive and negative work at different environment temperatures. Acta Physiol Scand 85:249, 1972
42. Nielsen B: Regulation of body temperature and heat dissipation at different levels of energy and heat production in man. Acta Physiol Scand 68:215, 1966
43. Nadel ER, Bergh U, Saltin B: Body temperature during negative work exercise. J Appl Physiol 33:553, 1972
44. Pahud P, Ravussin KJ, Acheson J, Jequiuer E: Energy expenditure during oxygen deficit of submaximal concentric and eccentric exercise. J Appl Physiol 49:16, 1980
45. Mannheimer JS: A comparison of strength gain between concentric and eccentric contractions. Phys Ther 49:1201, 1972
46. Jones A: The best kind of exercise. Iron Man 32:36, 1973
47. Johnson BL, Adamczyk JW, Tennoe KO, Stromme SB: A comparison of concentric and eccentric muscle training. Med Sci Sports 8:35, 1976
48. Johnson BL: Eccentric vs. concentric muscle training for strength development. Med Sci Sports 4:111, 1972
49. Newham DJ, McPhail G, Mills KR et al: Ultrastructural changes after concentric and eccentric contractions of human muscle. J Neurol Sci 61:109, 1983
50. Newham DJ, Mills KR, Quigley BM, Edwards RHT: Pain and fatigue after concentric and eccentric muscle contractions. Clin Sci 64:55, 1983
51. Eloranta V, Komi PV: Function of the quadriceps femoris muscle under maximal concentric and eccentric contractions. Electroencephalogr Clin Neurophysiol 20:159, 1980
52. Hendriksson J, Knuttgen HG, Bonde-Peterson F: Perceived exertion during exercise with concentric and eccentric muscle contractions. Ergonomics 15:537, 1972
53. Bonde-Peterson F, Hendriksson J, Knuttgen HG: Effect of training with eccentric muscle contractions on skeletal muscle metabolites. Acta Physiol Scand 88:564, 1973
54. Abbott BC, Bigland B, Ritchie JM: The physiological cost of negative work. J Physiol 117:380, 1952
55. Asmussen E, Hansen O, Lammert O: The relation between isometric and dynamic muscle strength in man. Communications of the Danish national association for infantile paralysis, 1965
56. Komi PV, Buskirk ER: Effect of eccentric and concentric muscle conditioning on tension and electrical activity in human muscle. Med Sci Sports Exerc 8:224, 1973
57. Jorgensen KL: Force-velocity relationships in human elbow flexors and extensors. In Komi PV (ed): Biomechanics V-A. University Park Press, Baltimore, 1976
58. Walmsley RP, Pearson N, Stymiest P: Eccentric wrist extensor contractions and the force velocity relationship in muscle. J Orthop Sports Phys Ther 8:288, 1986
59. Hageman PA, Gillaspie DM, Hill LD: Effects of speed and limb dominance on eccentric and concentric isokinetic testing of the knee. J Orthop Sports Phys Ther 10:59, 1988
60. Hart DL, Miller LC, Stauber WT: Effect of cooling on force oscillations during maximal voluntary eccentric exercise. Exp Neurol 90:73, 1985
61. Patton HD, Sundstein JW, Crill WE, Swanson PD: Introduction to Basic Neurology. WB Saunders, Philadelphia, 1976
62. Norman RW, Komi PV: Electro-mechanical delay in skeletal muscle under normal movement conditions. Acta Physiol Scand 106:241, 1979
63. Richmond FJR, Abrahams VC: Morphology and distribution of muscle spindles in dorsal muscles of the cat neck. J Neurophysiol 38:1322, 1975
64. Friden J, Seger J, Sjostrom M et al: Adaptive response in human skeletal muscle subjected to prolonged eccentric training. Int J Sports Med 4:177, 1983
65. Bocco C, Ito A, Komi PV et al: Neuromuscular function and mechanical efficiency of human leg extensor muscles during jumping exercises. Acta Physiol Scand 114:543, 1982

66. Bennett JG, Stauber WT: Evaluation and treatment of anterior knee pain using eccentric exercise. Med Sci Sports Exerc 18:528, 1986
67. Moritani T, DeVries HA: Neural factors versus hypertrophy in the time course of muscle strength gain. Am J Phys Med 58:115, 1979
68. Parmiggiani F, Stein RB: Non-linear summation of contractions in cat muscles. II. Later facilitation and stiffness changes. J Gen Physiol 78:295, 1981
69. Johnson MA, Polgar J, Weightman D, Appleton D: Data on the distribution of fibre types in thirty-six human muscles: an autopsy study. J Neurol Sci 18:111, 1973

3

Eccentrics: Clinical Program Design and Delayed Onset Muscle Soreness

CLINICAL PROGRAM DESIGN AND DECISION MAKING

In any rehabilitation program, a compromise is required between aggressive muscle overload techniques and safety/protection concerns. Eccentrics possesses potential for muscular/connective tissue damage and, clinically, measures will be taken to avoid or at least minimize resulting delayed onset muscle soreness (DOMS).

In the first half of this chapter we review considerations of eccentric training responses, describe advantages of eccentrics in specific clinical or performance applications, and examine proposed concepts of integrating eccentrics into the total rehabilitation plan. We do not suggest using eccentric training exclusively, but rather propose the use of eccentric biased exercise at the appropriate time.

Empirical evidence suggests that eccentrics is instituted after the subacute stage of inflammation has been achieved and follows successful tolerance of isometric and some concentric training. A phased, progressively demanding exercise continuum (Table 3-1) provides a guideline for initiating eccentrics. Of course, soft tissue healing constraints and related time periods present additional important guidelines to determine when eccentrics should be used.

The key variables of effective exercise applications are duration, intensity, frequency, and cycling of the sessions. *Cycling* refers to duration of training periods as it pertains to rest or tapering schedules. Quantified documentation of each of these varibles is vital to the assessment and problem solving of the subject's tolerance, progress toward goals, and identification and remediation of training plateaus.

Table 3-1. Davies Exercise Continuum

Multiple angle isometrics (submaximal effort)
Multiple angle isometrics (maximal)
Short arc concentric isokinetics (submaximal)
Short arc isotonics
Short arc concentric isokinetics (maximal)
Full ROM concentric isokinetics (submaximal)
Full ROM isotonics
Full ROM concentric isokinetics (maximal)

Abbreviation: ROM, range of motion.

TIMING OF CLINICAL APPLICATIONS

The clinical setting offers a variety of equipment and techniques to produce eccentric loads (Table 3-2). The appropriate timing of eccentric loading is therefore dependent on the type of technique used. In general, eccentric loads with slow joint speeds (defined as less than 120 degrees per sec-

Table 3-2. Clinical Sources of Eccentric Loading

Pulley stacks, free weights
Standard cam isotonic machines
Elastic bands
PNF, manual resistance
Controlled functional training
Robotics
Plyometrics
Treadmill
Impulse

Abbreviations: PNF, proprioceptive neuromuscular facilitation.

ond) are the first and least stressful selections. An exception to this rule is loading from the Impulse inertial unit (see Ch. 5).

Walsmley et al.[1] suggest that eccentrics should not be used for 30 hours postinjury and should be initiated when pain-free concentrics is achieved. They also mention waiting until near normal concentric strength levels have been reached, which we will demonstrate is overly cautious and not consistent with earliest return to function.

Depending on the degree of injury and success or type of treatment for inflammation, the subacute phase should be achieved in 3 to 7 days. Submaximal, slow speed eccentrics is started in the subactue period in balance with necessary soft tissue healing constraints. Collagen maturation proceeds in progressive fashion, with moderate tensile strength established in 3 weeks.[2] Early strength changes or gains (in the first 3 weeks) can be rapid and dramatic, while prolonged strength changes are gradual and represent structural or morphologic adaptations in muscle[3] (Fig. 3-1).

Mannheimer[4] concluded that eccentrics produced greater strengthening effects than concentrics only during the first 19 days after trauma, perhaps describing a differential effect on the neuromuscular system.

SETTING APPROPRIATE LOADS OR FORCES

Decisions about acceptable loads or forces with eccentric training are dependent on many patient factors, including, but not limited to, age, gender,

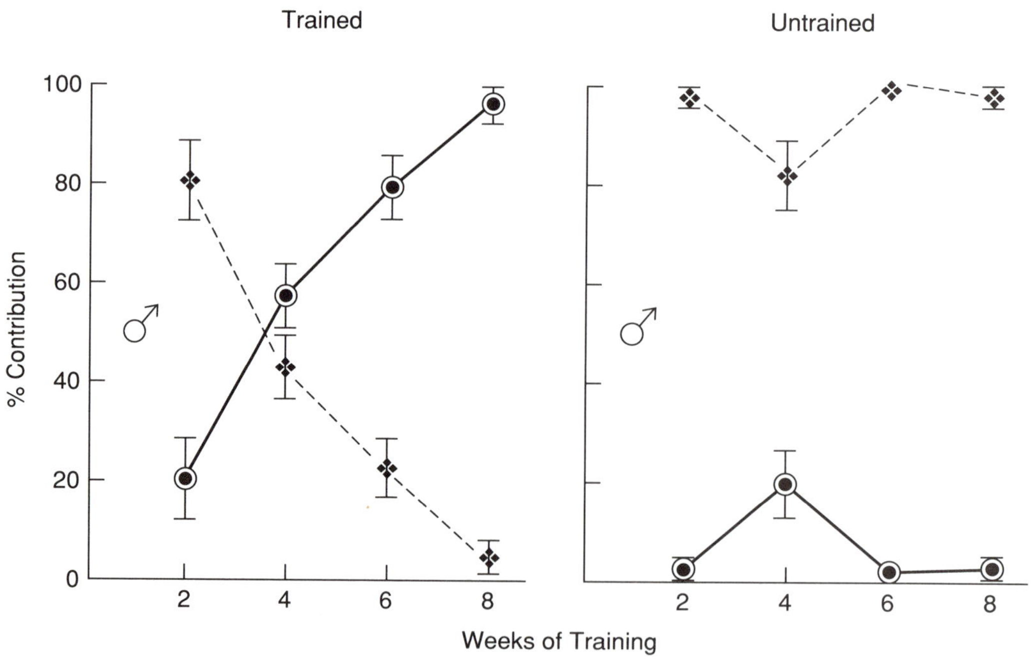

Fig. 3-1. Early neurologic versus morphologic changes in strength. (From Moritani and DeVries,[3] with permission.)

type and stage of injury or surgery, and previous physical training. Such decisions can be categorized into four general phases.

Phase I eccentric loading requires caution, with use of resistance in the form of limb weight and interactive gravitational forces only. During this period training includes a concentric phase for the target limb, with subsequent self-assisted eccentric (or negative) movement. If this approach is not well tolerated by the subject, or if poor control is evident (i.e., muscular shaking), the therapist or trainer may need to guide the negative phase. Phase I will usually be completed within 3 or fewer sessions, considering the goal of a controlled eccentric release of the involved limb without assisted movement.

Phase II progresses to submaximal loaded eccentrics with many available devices (i.e., elastic bands, machines, or free weights). This phase also includes training on the Impulse system. Johnson and Adamczyk[5] report safety to connective tissue and joint structures when eccentric training loads exceed the 1 repetition maximum (RM) concentric isotonic level by up to 20 percent, while loads between 20 to 40 percent greater than concentric 1 RM are risky. Loads in excess of 40 percent over the concentric capacity would be contraindicated. Hence, the clinical formula, eccentric training load = 120 percent of the 1 RM concentric load, provides a useful starting point for initial resisted work. Johnson and Adamczyk also propose a guideline for the suggested speed of the eccentric phase during early isotonics that takes at least 1 second to complete. During this phase, isolated eccentrics against a load are easily applied on cam and pulley type weight machines by exclusive use of the noninvolved limb for concentrics.

Phase III is generally the longest phase and corresponds to the patient's return to selected activities of daily living (ADL) or sport functional skills on a graded, controlled basis (Table 3-3). Intensity of loads are increased using systems such as Knight's daily adjusted progressive resistive exercise (DAPRE) plan.[6] The major change in training in this phase is the emphasis on involved-leg-only eccentrics, which in turn leads to submaximal closed chain exercise and use of functional eccentric progressions. Phase IV details are outlined in Table 3-3. Currently, lower extremity functional eccentric progressions are more commonly used

Table 3-3. Time-Phased Eccentric Training Progression

PHASE I	7–21 days 2 legged/arm concentric and eccentric motion Submaximal isotonics
PHASE II	7–21 days Open chain submaximal isotonics 2 legged/arm concentrics, injured limb only eccentric High mass impulse Submaximal, slow speed robotics
PHASE III	21–35 days Maximal effort open chain isotonic machines Closed chain isotonic machines Free weights Low mass impulse Robotics Initial level functional eccentrics leading to plyometrics
PHASE IV	21–50 days Closed chain maximal eccentrics Maximal robotics High stress functional eccentrics Plyometrics progressions (Many patients or types of problems will not progress to or require this phase.)

The suggested times are projections only, with actual days determined by patient variables and types of dysfunction.

and, therefore, have greater sophistication than corresponding upper extremity programs. A sample functional eccentric lower extremity progression would be structured as follows:

Stage 1. One-legged step-up onto 12-inch stool: noninvolved leg steps up first and down last
Stage 2. One-legged step up: involved leg steps up first, noninvolved leg steps down first
Stage 3. Repeat stage 1 with 18-inch step height
Stage 4. Repeat stage 2 with 18-inch step height
Stage 5. Slow quarter squats (Fig. 3-2)
Stage 6. Rapid quarter squats
Stage 7. Slow parallel squats (Fig. 3-3)
Stage 8. Rapid parallel squats

Stage 8 may be contraindicated in some types of knee dysfunction and all stages past 4 warrant careful thought about potential of joint structure irritation of injury.

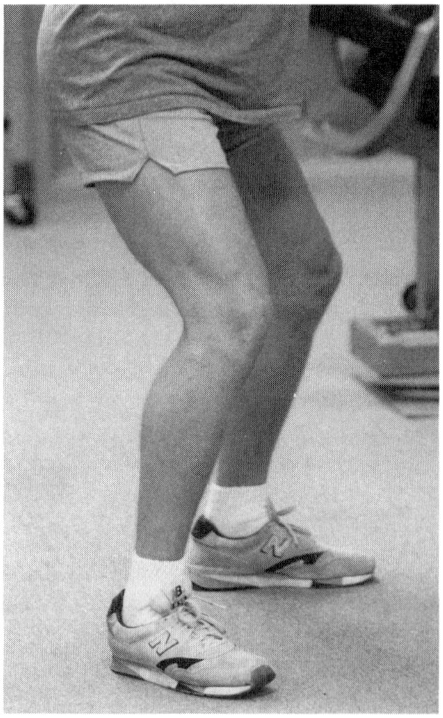

Fig. 3-2. Quarter squat position (knees flexed to approximately 30 degrees).

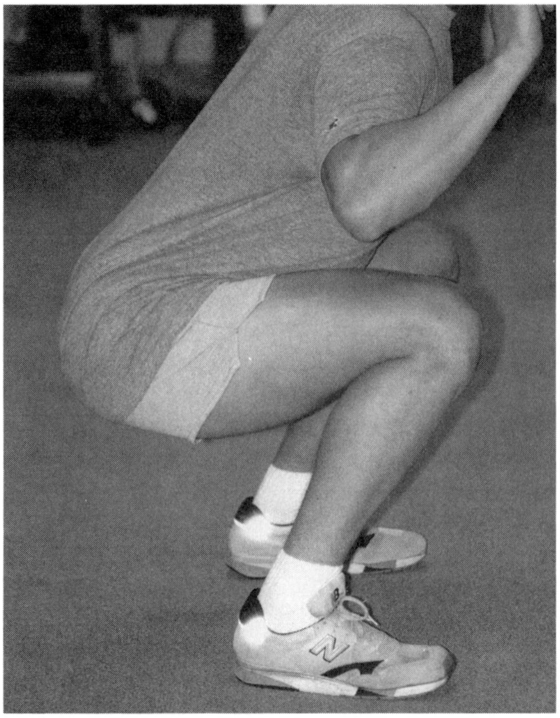

Fig. 3-3. Parallel squat position.

A well-developed and carefully phased eccentric program has been outlined by Curwin and Stanish.[7] Although they designed the program specifically for tendonitis problems, it has equally sound applications for other indications with eccentric training. The program combines the effects of load and speed of movement to set the resulting eccentric forces in an incremental, gradual manner that is reviewed in Figure 3-4. This example of a "drop and stop" program includes the clinically important concept of increasing speed by asking the patient to move through a set arc or range of motion (ROM); for example, 90 degrees in the case of the knee, in a shorter period. A clinical method to control and monitor the length of the eccentric phase time involves going from a 4-count basis to a 1-count basis for the same ROM, which corresponds roughly to a 1.5-second eccentric period with the 4 count and .25 to .3 sec-

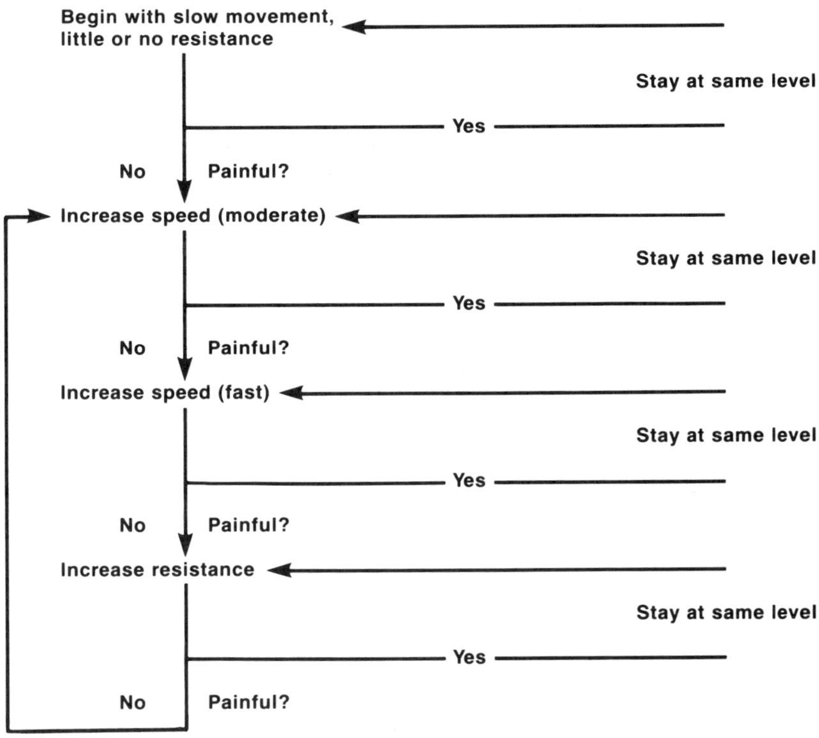

Fig. 3-4. Outline of eccentric exercise program for tendonitis. (From Curwin and Stanish,[7] with permission.)

onds (250 to 300 milliseconds) for the 1 count for a 90 degree arc of motion.

One example of a functionally based, eccentric upper extremity progression is the developmental scheme for the return to throwing outlined by Blackburn.[8] This throwing program uses a progressively demanding biomechanical design to incorporate decreased distance with corresponding increased velocity of throws to the demands of pitching. The rotator cuff and related muscles are recruited to effectively decelerate the arm at increased velocities, thereby causing increased eccentric demands. The key with upper extremity eccentric progressions is the selective recruitment of the rotator cuff muscles in a synergistic, coordinated pattern of use prior to any diagonal or overhead types of motions. As additional approaches to upper extremity programs are developed and verified as effective, consideration of both open and closed kinetic chain emphasis will be beneficial.

SETTING SETS, REPETITIONS, AND REST PERIODS

Fifteen years ago, Johnson and Adamczyk[5] identified the need for additional research on repetitions, sets, and rest periods, yet the current knowledge on this topic remains uncertain. Due to the low oxygen requirement with eccentric muscle responses, rest periods between training bouts need not be prolonged. Although the literature does not specify optimal rest periods, Laycoe and Marteniuk[9] adopted a 1-minute rest period between eccentric training phases. Clinical experience dictates that 30 seconds to 1 minute is sufficient to permit controlled repeat sets within the tolerance levels of almost all types of patients or dysfunctions. Varied training regimens with sets and repetitions have been presented,[5–13] with no study using more than 3 sets. However, suggested repetitions range from 3 maximal effort up to 20 repetitions.[11,12] In summary, optimal strengthening effects appear to be gained in a maximum of 3 sets containing from 3 to 20 repetitions. Future studies on optimal repetitions and training effectiveness should consider the differential effects of training speed, type of muscle loading (isotonic versus isokinetic), and specific muscle groups.

In view of the known recovery period of 3 to 7 days after DOMS, frequency of eccentric training sessions is advisable no more than 3 times per week. Studies that used 4 training sessions per week, demonstrated either minimal strength improvement (2.9 percent per week),[11] or actual decreases in force production.[13] In fact, the physiologic process of DOMS resolution dictates the safest frequency to be only 2 times per week. With the clinical standard of muscle training being 3 times per week, usually on a Monday, Wednesday, and Friday basis, two options exist for eccentric training plans. The first plan would be to administer heavy eccentric training on Monday and Friday. Due to patient schedule constraints or needs to integrate other clinical treatment measures, a staggered schedule such as Monday–Friday–Wednesday–Monday (then repeated) is an alternative.

Continued research on the optimal parameters of eccentric training programs is warranted and future eccentric applications depend on upgraded knowledge bases to ensure both improved results and the prevention or decrease of DOMS.

AGE AND GENDER ISSUES WITH ECCENTRIC TRAINING

Current physiologic and clinical literature indicate potentially significant differences between young subjects and older subjects, as well as between male and females; in responses to eccentric muscle loads. Specificity of eccentric training programs along these lines will provide safer and perhaps accelerated results.

Griffin[14] proposed that the differences between eccentric and concentric force capacities of a single muscle, the so-called eccentric to concentric force ratio, was less pronounced in females, as determined by isokinetic tests. Trudelle-Jackson et al.[15] also reported a consistent depression of eccentric to concentric quadriceps ratios in normal young females and raised the issue of a potential predisposition to certain types of knee dysfunction as a corollary. If this observation is consistent across age and activity variables, an important clinical result may be that females will respond more optimally with eccentric biased training than males. Such differential training responses may be related to viscoelastic considerations or time-based neuromuscular adaptations. It has also been reported that women demonstrate less marked enzyme releases in response to exercise than men.[16,17]

Highenboten et al.[18] observed that normal subjects aged 15 to 24 years produced significantly higher concentric torque values for quadriceps and hamstrings than subjects aged 25 to 34 years. However, the torque differences for eccentrics between the two age groups were minimal. Thus, if a similar relationship exists for older groups, a selective benefit of eccentric biased training with older subjects may be an important rehabilitation approach. Certainly, several clear advantages of eccentric training with elderly patients are apparent in the areas of exercise tolerance and motivation. Many elderly patients presenting for either neurologic or orthopedic rehabilitation programs are deconditioned from both a cardiorespiratory and muscular standpoint and may have images of rehabilitation as a threatening or painful endeavor. Often, the use of concentric resistive exercise is poorly tolerated in the initial phases of their rehabilitation programs. Due to the cycle of pain during or after exercise, many patients fail to progress with additional weight increases and have difficulty performing appropriate breathing mechanics. They also develop strong negative reinforcement patterns that interfere with eventual program outcome and delay the time to recovery. Due to the efficiency of eccentric muscle responses related to low oxygen requirement and the lower perception of effort per level of muscular tension, eccentric training provides an ideal alternative to many problems associated with elderly patients. Also, because of their ability to safely and comfortably achieve much higher weight or force levels with eccentrics than had been possible previously, many patients are provided a concrete positive reinforcement; with such a small success, the overall motivational level and corresponding compliance factors are suddenly and dramatically increased.

Another observation of elderly intolerance to early exercise approaches relates to the consistent difficulty that is encountered with isometric contractions. Isometric exercises are often poorly executed and commonly forgotten soon after instruction and practice sessions. Furthermore, isometric exercises raise the potential for valsalva conditions, which are poorly tolerated by many elderly patients. The electromyographic (EMG) study by Andrew[19] identified isometrics as an effective muscular training method for patients who are unable to activate muscle due to pain or neurologic impairment (both commonly seen in elderly patients) and found little difference in muscular tension levels between isometrics and eccentrics. An altered neuromuscular control that interferes with normal skeletal muscle relaxation is a possible explanation for the isometric contraction difficulties experienced by the elderly. This loss of control may correspond to the equivalent of constant low level EMG activity in the target muscle. Thus, submaximal eccentrics may provide an effective substitute for isometrics as the initial phase of a time-based exercise continuum that prepares the patient for more strenuous resistance modes in a progressive manner.

With respect to the growing percentage of the population and number of persons aged 65 years or older and the need for skillful and frequent physical rehabilitation, continued research regarding the specific and unique effects of eccentric training for the elderly is both promising and warranted.

GENERAL ECCENTRIC PROGRAM PRINCIPLES AND PERSPECTIVES

Clinical program design for eccentrics must be based on key principles of physiologic differences, safety concepts, and training variables that can optimize goals and results. Specific training effects are dependent on the interaction of limb position, velocity of movement, type of contraction, joint angle, and parameters used.[20] A current concept in the scientific literature involves the quantification of expected muscular strength changes associated with various types or modes of muscle loading.

Studies on the time course of strength gains for isokinetics are very consistent.[21–23] Cote et al.[21] determined an increase in isokinetic torque of the quadriceps muscle of 5 percent per week, while Grimby et al.[22] and Thomee et al.[23] described a .7 percent per week increase (4.9 percent) in the same muscle. Despite possible limitations in generalizing these results to other upper or lower extremity muscle groups, a clinically useful guideline is presented in these studies. As a point of reference, the program results from eccentric biased training are more variable. Singh and Karpovich[11] described a 2.9 percent increase in strength of the forearm extensors per week, Johnson et al.[24] reported 5.9 percent per week increase in quadriceps and a 5.3 percent per week increase in the biceps brachii, and Laycoe and Marteniuk[9] reported the largest weekly strength increase in the literature of 6.9 percent in the quadriceps muscle. It should be mentioned that Johnson et al.[24] studied four different upper and lower extremity muscle groups and determined no significant superiority of either concentric or eccentric biased training on weekly strength gains.

My personal clinical experience with intensive isotonic, free weight training over variable time periods has consistently identified the maximal weekly strength gain to be 5 percent per week. Eccentric biased strength training (see Ch. 7) is associated with muscular strength and power increases as well as prominent hypertrophy. This hypertrophy (equivalent to increase of muscular cross-sectional area) has been widely believed to be caused primarily by alterations in skeletal muscle proteins of the myofiber. However, due to concurrent responses in fibroblastic activity during eccentric training, the actual hypertrophy may be caused by increased thickness or density of the fascial and series elastic components (SEC) within the muscle.[25] Therefore, eccentric type training may not have any greater effect in enlarging muscle cell size than other types of dynamic exercise modes.

Another clinically important feature of eccentric muscle training involves the effects on subsequent development of DOMS. Performance of limited eccentric exercise (as little as a single bout) has been demonstrated to produce an adaptation that resists further DOMS symptoms.[26–28] Although eccentric training causes an ongoing cycle of muscular damage and repair,[25] the second exposure to eccentrics results in a reduced response, called the *repeated bout effect* by Clarkson et al.[27]. The repeated bout effect has been demonstrated for both upper and lower extremity muscle groups as well as for different activities and sports.[26–30] It is apparent that minimal training exposure to eccentrics can produce a relative immunity to DOMS damage for as much as 6 weeks[26] and enzyme leakage for at least 1 week.[31] Although the mechanism of this important effect is unclear, Armstrong[31] and Byrnes et al.[32] suggest that the first bout of eccentric tension serves to destroy certain stress-susceptible muscle fibers (perhaps type II) that cause DOMS; repeated bouts would therefore damage fewer susceptible fibers with a correspondent reduction of symptoms.

Furthermore, eccentric muscle training offers several potential advantages with respect to physiologic overflow of training effects. Eccentrics may cause overflow across speeds to antagonistic muscles of the trained muscle, and to other forms of muscle loads (i.e., concentrics). In fact, Singh and Karpovich[11] found training effects from eccentric training to be greater in the untrained antagonsitic muscles than in the trained muscle. Disagreement about overflow from one exercise type to another (mode specificity) is prevalent in the literature. While Chandler and Duncan[33] and Nicely et al.[34] reported that eccentric training is mode specific with normal quadriceps muscle, Ellenbecker et al.[35] determined the overflow effects of eccentric training to concentric torque to be greater than the opposite interaction. Tomberlin and Basford[36] also reported eccentric strength training overflow to concentrics, but the effect was limited to men. As suggested by Duncan et al.,[10] the lack of physiologic carryover or overflow from eccentrics to concentrics could be caused by the minimal fatigue effects of high speed eccentric training and a corresponding need to incorporate higher repetitions to produce fatigue.

With isokinetic eccentric (robotics or active) studies, overflow across different joint speeds has been demonstrated. While Walmsley et al.[1] stated that eccentric training was velocity specific, Duncan et al.[10] demonstrated overflow of 60 degrees per second above and below the training speed and suggested the possibility of overflow to a greater speed range than their data examined.

Due to the heat production associated with intense or prolonged eccentric loads, it is advisable to provide a convenient source of drinking water for the patient during and following the eccentric sessions. An increase in body temperature will lead to rapid sweat responses in most patients, and consideration should be made of the individual's thermoregulatory capacity, including past history of heat illness and current medical conditions. For example, the debilitated patient, often with low motivational status concerning vigorous exercise, presents a dual challenge for the health professional. Due to low cardiorespiratory reserves, such a patient is better suited to eccentric resistance training, but may not tolerate this type of loading approach due to body temperature changes and sweat responses.

The appropriate positioning of an eccentric exercise bout within a single session is dependent on two factors: (1) sufficient increase in local body temperature, and (2) flexibility exercises to facilitate increased distensibility. These factors will ensure viscoelastic compliance in the working muscle areas. A general plan to safely integrate differ-

Table 3-4. Single Eccentric Training Session Structure (Suggested Integration with Other Exercise Modes)

General aerobic warm-up (example: Ube, Fitron)
Flexibility for target muscles (static)
Submaximal eccentric movement as a "cueing" effect
Isokinetics (if used)
General isotonics (if used)
Functional eccentric training bout
Cryotherapy

ent types of muscle loading and encourage optimal performance of each distinct type of exercise is reviewed in Table 3-4. This progression has been used for over 15 years with consistent success in varied orthopedic and sports settings. However, additional research on optimal program design features is greatly needed.

ECCENTRIC PROGRAM INDICATIONS AND CASE STUDIES

Successful program planning will depend on the specific biomechanical requirements of various activities or sports and the biomechanics involved in a particular injury mechanism. Several biomechanical perspectives are reviewed in the literature and provide the clinician with a starting point for eccentric programs.

Studies of the knee joint demostrate specific biomechanical indications for eccentric training that are dependent on the joint position. Arms et al.[37] describe the use of eccentric knee extension at a 45 degree flexed position to reduce strain in the anterior cruciate ligament (ACL). Use of this biomechanical principle has promising applications for the protracted rehabilitation required after ACL reconstruction surgery. Lieb and Perry[38] identify the first 15 degrees of eccentric knee flexion as the most difficult to control due to joint arthrokinematics and length-tension factors of the quadriceps. Stanton and Purdam[20] report a highly specific rehabilitation protocol for the hamstrings using a hip/knee positional interaction similar to that used during running, with emphasis on high speed eccentric muscular "catches" (Figs. 3-5 and 3-6). Walking gait determinants and related muscular demands for hip abduction were investigated by Olson et al.[39] They concluded that rapid, eccentric hip abduction tension was required between 20 to 40 degrees of hip abduction for normal gait and that eccentric muscular training was important to both normal tension development as well as neuromuscular re-education. The final specific application of eccentric muscular demands involves the spine. Although additional EMG, biomechanical, ergonometric, and clinical studies are indicated, the position of function for the low back

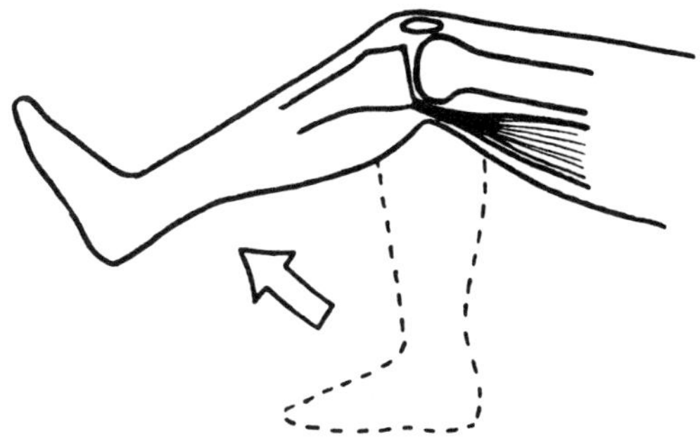

Fig. 3-5. Quick active knee extension is rapidly decelerated at 20 to 30 degrees via eccentric hamstring contraction. This is followed by a quick concentric contraction. (From Stanton and Purdam,[20] with permission.)

appears to be from 10 degrees of hyperextension to 45 degrees of flexion.[40,41] Jackson and Brown[41] determined that the key role of the lumbar extensors in the eccentric mode was to stabilize the body for postural demands such as lowering the trunk during bending and lifting. Future rehabilitation for the lumbar spine may benefit from eccentric training principles, whereas discharge planning and risk profiles may benefit from an improved understanding of concentric/eccentric torque relationships for the lumbar extensors.

Yet another key indication for the selective use of eccentric muscular training concerns the re-

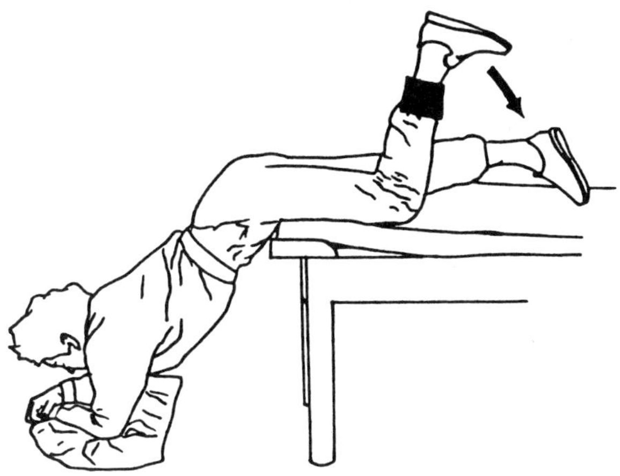

Fig. 3-6. "Catch" exercise performed laying prone over the edge of a bed. (From Stanton and Purdam,[20] with permission.)

mediation of strength plateaus that may develop during extended training or rehabilitation programs. Plateaus in strength or force development are frustrating to the training professional and client alike. Such periods of minimal changes in strength, despite continued and many times disciplined, structured training may be caused by several variables, acting separately or in combination. First, plateaus may be caused by normal variations in strength.[42,43] Another possibility described by Pavone and Moffat[44] is the biomechanical disruption caused by inappropriate length-tension principles in the working musculature and arthrokinematic difficulties in the target joint(s). The final explanation for plateaus includes the concept of overtraining, or staleness. Over training possesses both biochemical and psychological attributes.

Eccentric biased training techniques offer a useful method to remediate all of the causes of strength plateaus, including the attributes of overtraining. With overtraining presentations, efficiency of eccentrics and altered psychological perception of effort promote a fresh alternative for improved motivation. Table 3-5 reviews other clinical areas that are indications for the selective use of eccentric training programs.

The following two case studies were selected on the basis of successful outcomes with eccentric biased training, minimal use of confounding variables (e.g., modalities, prolonged rest periods, or contributory history) and relatively short time periods to return to normal functional activities. In most therapeutic settings, success is measured with the simple formula of brief time periods relative to the type of dysfunction and the resolution of symptoms and resumption of desired or necessary functional activities.

Table 3-5. Clinical Indications for Eccentric Biased Exercise

Mechanical, reproducible joint pain
Joint pain resistant to modality treatments
Unidirectional joint crepitus or pain arc
Deconditioned or patients with low endurance
Plateaus in strength gains
Low motivated patient
Tendonitis presentations
Late stage rehabilitation and performance training

CASE 1

Patient Description: Eighty-two year-old white woman in good general health, who is married and drives herself.

Admitting Diagnosis: Referring physician speciality: neruologist. Diagnosis: distal neuropathy with proximal weakness.

History and Chief Complaint: Following a one week bout in bed with an upper respiratory infection, the patient noticed pain in the bilateral quadriceps during walking and prolonged standing (over 10 minutes) and weakness of bilateral lower extremities during ascent/descent of stairs or curbs. The patient also experienced an inability to rise from chairs without assistance from her husband. This particular functional problem led her to visit an orthopedist, who in turn referred her to a neurologist. The patient reported no previous pain or functional problems like she was currently experiencing.

Contributory History: Patient had increased upper thoracic kyphosis with typical "dowager's hump" deformity, as well as episodic pain, stiffness, and muscle spasms in this area.

Physical Examination Results: Neurologic examination: within normal limits (WNL). Bilateral active ROM for hips, knees, and ankles were WNL with respect to age considerations. Bilateral quadriceps setting control was fair. (*Fair* is defined as ability to actively, isometrically contract quadriceps with sufficient force to move the patella superiorly, but not with firm vastus medialis obliquus control.)

Manual muscle tests
Quadriceps, R/L, 4/4 −
Hamstrings, R/L, 5 − /4
Hip flexion, R/L, 5 − /4
Hip extension, R/L, 4/4 +
Hip abduction, R/L, 3 + /3 +
Active straight leg raise (flexibility)
R/L, 50 degrees/79 degrees

Impression: An insidious onset of bilateral muscular weakness of the antigravity muscles and bilateral hamstring inflexibility, causing biomechanical gait dysfunction and functional deficits.

Program Structure: The patient was instructed in home program exercises as follows:

Supine hip extension (knees flexed, feet flat), 3 sets of 10
Hip abduction straight leg raises, 3 sets of 10
Supine hamstring stretch, 1 minute hold
Step-ups onto large phone book, 3 sets of 3

On the second visit, the following additions/adjustments were made:

Step-ups onto two phone books, 3 sets of 5; alternating with left foot up first, left foot down first; repeated with right foot in the same order
Discontinuation of supine hip extension due to onset of upper back tightness and aching pain
Quarter level squats with chair used for balance and assistance (corresponding to a 30-degree knee flexion angle)

On the third visit, the patient demonstrated good compliance with home program and overall tolerance of all exercises. The following addition was made:

Parallel squats with chair used for guidance and assistance to concentric phase, 3 sets of 5

On the fourth and final visit, the patient was carefully instructed in the importance of continuing home exercises for at least 1 month, 3 times per week.

Program Results: The patient's thigh pain during walking/standing gradually resolved in sessions 1 to 3, with the weakness experienced on curbs, stairs, and rising from a chair resolving entirely by the fourth visit. The patient had resumed full, normal ADL with complete independence at discharge. The total time from admittance to the program to discharge was 20 days, during which there were 4 visits. By the fourth visit, her upper thoracic muscular pain had also resolved.

CASE 2

Patient Description: Twenty-five-year-old white man in excellent general health.

Admitting Diagnosis and Chief Complaint: The patient experienced a sudden, stabbing pain in his right anterior knee during a high speed, lunging motion in a racquetball game. Despite use of ice on the knee after the game, the patient experienced increased pain later in the day and pronounced stiffness and pain the following morning. Diagnosis: acute strain in the right infrapatellar tendon.

Contributory History: The patient was a former collegiate gymnast who routinely ran 2 to 3 times per week and played competitive racquetball 3 to 4 times per week. The patient reported no previous knee dysfunction.

Physical Examination Results: Slight tenderness of infrapatellar pole and tendon, with no swelling noted. All lower extremity strengths were WNL with the exception of the right knee extension, grade 4+ with increased pain. There was slight restriction of passive prone knee flexion, R/L-130 degrees/140 degrees. Lower extremity postural alignment was also WNL.

Impression: Due to focal involvement of the right infrapatellar tendon, minimal findings despite the acute pain, as well as the distinct biomechanical cause of an uncontrolled, eccentric loading moment, a gradually progressive, eccentric biased program was indicated.

Program Structure: In the first session (the day after injury) the patient was instructed in and treated with static, prone knee flexion stretch to tolerance for 1 minute 2 times per day, treated with ice massage to the point of skin anesthesia, also 2 times per day; and started on an isotonic (Nautilus) negative eccentric (negatives) program with a starting level of 3 plates, executed with a two-legged concentric and eccentric phase at a moderate speed. The weight level was selected by the maximal weight that was controlled in a pain-free manner. Session 2 differed only in the use of

2 plates on the isotonics, with two-legged concentric, followed by *injured leg only* eccentrics. Sessions 3 and 4 progressed to 3 plates with the same sequence. All isotonics were done on the basis of 3 sets of 10 repetitions.

Program Results: The patient was discharged on the fourth session because of extended travel plans and the complete resolution of tenderness or pain with all activities, except racquetball. The patient was advised to resume racquetball gradually, cautioned to warm up with flexibility exercises prior to play, and told to ice the area after. The patient did resume full competitive racquetball with no recurrence of symptoms one week after discharge. The total time from admission to return to full competition was 11 days.

DELAYED ONSET MUSCULAR SORENESS

Post-exercise soreness, also known as delayed onset muscle soreness (DOMS) and delayed muscle soreness (DMS), is widely reported[25,45,46] to occur as a consequence of eccentric muscle loading 24 to 48 hours after the exercise bout. It is not associated with concentric-only types of exercise.[47–49] DOMS may result from as few as 15 repetitions[50] and gentle eccentric loads in the untrained subject. Symptoms may last up to 1 week, with most cases being resolved in 72 hours.[45] Symptom intensity generally peaks at 48 hours.

The symptom cluster of DOMS includes pain (or soreness) of a dull, diffuse nature[51] with varible intensity depending on the relative overload stimulus for a given individual's neuro-musculotendinous system (Table 3-6). Other symptoms include stiffness, that which is perceived both during stretch of the involved muscle and during isometric contractions in a shortened position of the involved muscle,[45] and tenderness. *Tenderness* is defined as pain induced by direct pressure, and is commonly described as most intense in the distal lateral aspect of the quadriceps femoris muscle group.[12,45] Hasson et al.[12] report that as much as 40 to 50 percent of the total muscle area can be tender (Fig. 3-7).

The signs manifested in DOMS are consistent and include muscle swelling,[25,29] loss of active ROM,[47,52] and decreased peak active force potential of the involved muscle with corresponding alteration in EMG activity (i.e., EMG levels that are elevated above normal for a given muscle load). For example, Yackzan et al.[47] defined a 36.4 percent loss of elbow extension range at 48 hours postexercise, while Hasson et al.[12] reported decreases in isometric force of 33.4 percent and decreases in peak isokinetic torque 12.1 percent. Scientific literature is unclear regarding the influence of DOMS on passive ROM.

There are five general theories that attempt to explain the etiology and process of DOMS:

1. Lactic acid theory (Assmussen[53])
2. Torn tissue theory (Hough[54])
3. Tonic muscle spasms (DeVries[55])
4. Connective tissue damage (multiple investigators[53,56–59])
5. Tissue fluid theory (Stauber[25])

Each theory presents a version of either metabolic or mechanical chain reactions that manifest in the clinical syndrome of DOMS. Careful examination of the various theories and events with DOMS suggests an interdependent causation between many metabolic and mechanical disruptions (Fig. 3-8). In view of the nonlimiting influence of eccentric work on muscle circulation, the concentration of anaerobic end products, such as lactic acid, are minimal and cannot be expected to cause DOMS. The biochemical studies of

Table 3-6. Comparison of Three Modes of Exercise on Rating of Perceived Soreness and Serum CPK

	Rating of Perceived Soreness				Increase in CPK Activity
Exercise Mode	Pre	5 h	10 h	25 h	(%)
Eccentric	1.0	2.3	2.8	5.5	35.8
Isometric	1.0	1.5	1.4	3.2	34.0
Concentric	1.0	1.0	1.1	1.0	37.6

Abbreviation: CPK, creatine phosphokinase.
(From Clarkson et al.,[95] with permission.)

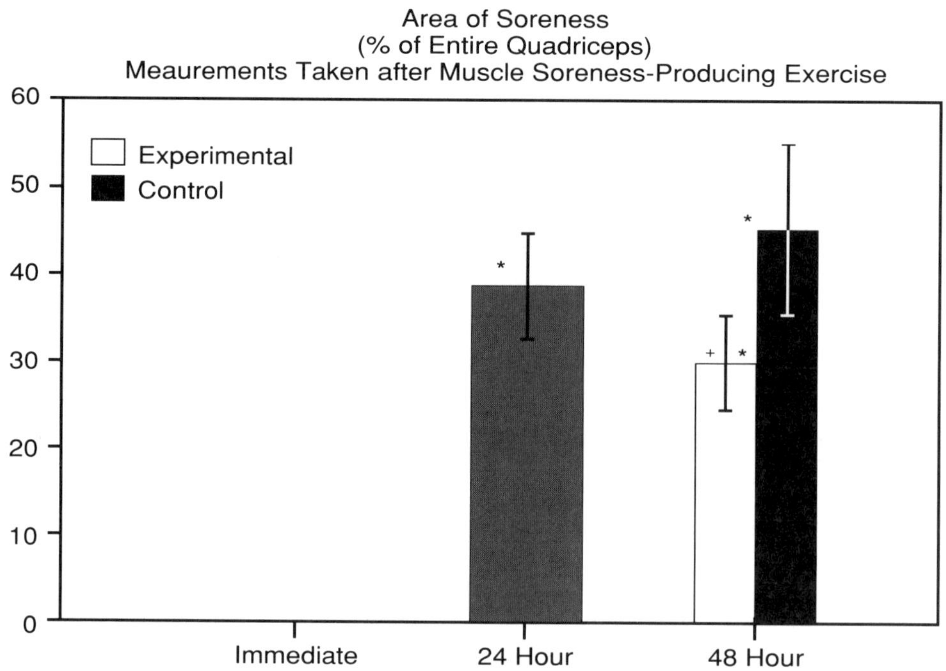

Fig. 3-7. Total area of muscle influenced by DOMS. Area of muscle soreness (expressed as a percentage of entire quadriceps). The data are reported as means ±SD, difference between baseline and other time measures. (+), the difference between experimental and control at 48 hours ($P < 0.05$).

Schwane et al.[60] and Waltrous et al.[61] have verified this relationship and therefore the lactic acid theory can be discounted. Friden and Sjostrom[62] however, raise the issue of a potential lactic acidosis role in the production of the observed Z-line degeneration that is a proven correlate of DOMS. In addition, the tonic spasm theory has also been discounted by EMG studies that were unable to demonstrate any increased activity in sore muscles.[63,64]

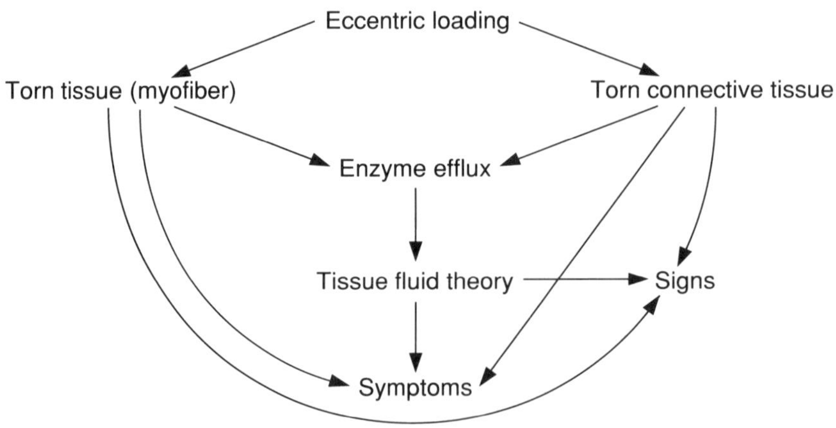

Fig. 3-8. Interaction of torn tissue and connective damage theories of DOMS.

TORN TISSUE THEORY

The torn tissue theory is supported by several studies[63,65–67] that trace biochemical markers of muscle injury such as myoglobin and describe the disruption of subcellular components such as the Z line, or disc. Friden[66] represents the Z line as the mechanically weakest link in the contractile machinery and characterizes myofibrillar damage as more dependent on peak tension than total average forces.

The majority of ultrastructural (subcellular) damage was found in type IIb fibers[66], which is consistent with Friden et al.'s[67] description of type IIb fibers having the narrowest or weakest Z bands. On a macroscopic level, Garrett and Duncan[68] described the weakest link of the muscle as the musculotendinous junction, while Newham et al.[45] demonstrated the greatest level of DOMS in the same area. The Z-line damage, apparent with microscopy as streaming or total disruption, is interpreted by Friden and Sjostrom[62] and Newham et al.[45] as rupturing of myofibrillar tissue with secondary releases of hydrolases and by Armstrong et al.[65] as inflammatory responses to degenerating fibers and macrophage infiltration.

The torn tissue theory also comprises such events as damage to the sarcoplasmic reticulum[45] and to the T tubule,[25] both of which interfere with normal calcium metabolism. Less calcium release per action potential may explain the observed fatigue to low frequency electrical stimulation.[45,69] Despite the limitations of studying mice, McCully and Faulkner[50] demonstrated that 37 percent of the total muscle fibers were damaged to various extents, while the first signs of regeneration appeared at 4 days postexercise.

TORN CONNECTIVE TISSUE THEORY

Selective damage from eccentrics to SEC (composed of the epimysium, perimysium, endomysium, fascia, and tendons) is widely supported.[13,63,70,71] Due to selective recruitment of fast twitch muscle fiber with eccentrics and the greater density of slow twitch fiber endomysium, fast twitch fibers appear highly susceptible to eccentric damage.[72] As mentioned in the previous section, disruption of the sarcoplasmic reticulum results in altered relaxation capacity of the contracting muscle, which in turn could cause a shear force between myofiber units at the level of the endomysium.[25,73] Tullson and Armstrong[70,71] reported the low hexose monophosphate shunt (HMS) activity resulting from eccentric loads as indicative of selective damage to the connective tissue as opposed to muscle. In addition, pain associated with DOMS can be explained by the location of group IV sensory fibers within the endomysium and fascia.[74–76]

ENZYME EFFLUX FROM ECCENTRIC LOADS

While both the torn tissue and torn connective tissue theories are consistent with the timing of soreness following eccentric loads, they both describe cellular damage that produces pronounced enzyme or protein degradation product release into the extracellular spaces. This "cascade" of collagen and protein metabolities is termed *efflux*,[66] and represents a "passing away."[77] The resultant enzyme efflux from eccentric muscle activity involves several key substances: hydroxyproline[63]; calcium ion[25,45,78]; creatine phosphokinase (CPK)[49,60,79,80]; and myoglobin.[53] The skeletal muscle enzyme efflux of these substances is proportional to the intensity and duration of the exercise and is less pronounced in females.[81] Enzyme efflux may be caused by two mechanisms: (1) altered membrane permeability and (2) fiber degeneration and necrosis.

Duncan[78] determined that the calcium ion produced muscular damage similar to that of eccentric exercise when in direct contact with muscle tissue. Thus, the question of whether calcium antagonist agents, such as verapamil, would be effective in preventing and/or treating exertional muscle damage, becomes worthy of investigation.[82]

When comparing running with cycling (with no eccentric phase), the magnitude of CPK[80] was increased 10- to 200-fold. Secondary to downhill running, Schwane et al.[60] demonstrated a 351 percent increase of CK at 24 hours postexercise and a 141 percent elevation above resting values at 48 hours. While CPK is related to soreness, Newham[79] concluded it could not actually cause DOMS because peak concentrations occurred as the soreness was resolving.

Although the underlying pathophysiology of DOMS remains unclear, it is interesting that the magnitude of CPK release is similar to that found in Duchenne muscular dystrophy and other syndromes of diseased muscle.[80]

TISSUE FLUID THEORY

It may be reasoned that the enzyme efflux during DOMS will establish a diffusion gradient for fluid across the cellular membrane into extracellular spaces that perpetuates continued swelling or edema. As described by Stauber[25], the pain and swelling of DOMS resembles a mini-compartment syndrome and the extracellular space may be considered to be of primary importance in the events of DOMS. Indeed, two studies found that tissue fluid pressure was elevated in muscles exercised eccentrically, but not concentrically.[83,84] This type of intramuscular, extracellular swelling was described by Howell et al.[29] in an analogy comparing the muscle with a water balloon stuffed inside a nylon stocking. Increased fluid volume inside the balloon would produce tension effects throughout the stocking with resulting pain, swelling, and stiffness. Hasson et al.[12] also support the presence of tissue edema as an element of DOMS and treatment with reciprocal, resisted exercise to produce the "muscle pump" effect on the fluid.

Future research aimed at clarifying the unique roles of torn tissue, torn connective tissue, and extracellular fluid mechanisms for DOMS is needed. While DOMS is a negative element of eccentric training, it may provide a tool to study the optimal intensity, frequency, and duration of eccentric muscle loading programs and the timing of treatment regimens for eccentric-induced musculotendinous damage.

TREATMENT FOR DOMS

The presence of reactive inflammation as a correlate of the pathophysiology of DOMS is a significant factor[12,25,47,48] and warrants attention for appropriate treatment strategies. However, inflammation was discounted by Schwane et al.[60] because of the absence of white blood cells or neutrophil increases. Despite support for the efficacy of cryotherapy in alleviating inflammation,[85–87] Yackzan et al.[47] found no effect of cryotherapy in preventing or alleviating the pain or functional problems associated with DOMS. The extent of inflammation in DOMS is therefore a controversial issue that deserves further research investigation.

A number of suggested treatments to facilitate the resolution of DOMS are listed in Table 3-7; because of minimal supporting evidence on the efficacy of any specific treatment technique, the list is by no means inclusive. In fact, many other types of treatment may prove to be successful or superior to those listed. Since prevention strategies are not presently available, several important questions arise when considering the treatment for DOMS. First, what is the relevance of treatment for DOMS if the condition is self-limited and resolves within 3 to 4 days? Does skillful neglect provide the optimal approach? Whether the patient is an athlete after an intense contest, a weekend recreational athlete, or a housewife after vigorous gardening, 3 to 4 days of lost time represent

Table 3-7. Suggested Treatment Techniques for DOMS

Type	Efficacy
Rest	None
Nonsteroidal anti-inflammatory[88]	Highly successful
Steroidal anti-inflammatory[89–91]	Moderately successful
Electrical stimulation[45]	Proposed only
Exercise[12,54,57]	Highly successful
TENS[92,93]	Highly successful
Stretching[55,94]	Mixed success
Iontophoresis[12]	Not successful
Cryotherapy[47]	Not successful
Calcium antagonists[82]	Proposed only

Abbreviation: TENS, transcutaneous electrical nerve stimulation.

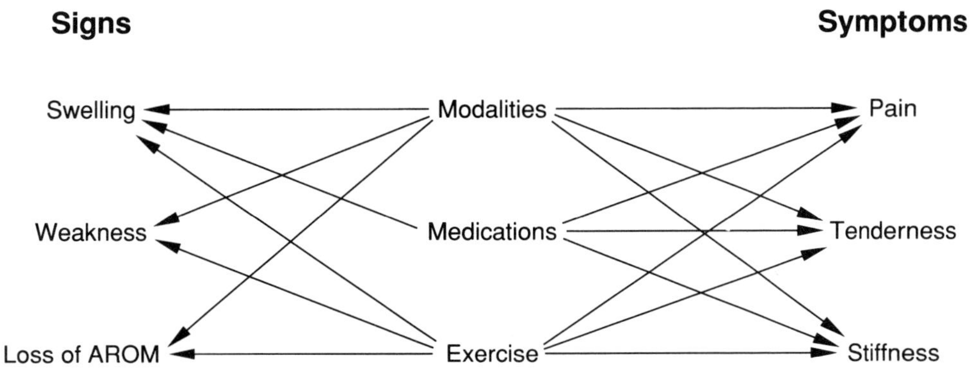

Fig. 3-9. Paradigm for DOMS treatment.

significant problems that warrant effective intervention techniques. However, what should the timing of treatment after eccentric training be? What is the effect of singular treatment modes versus a program of combined treatments?

It seems logical to base treatment on both biomechanical and biochemical areas, with selection from three basic options: medications or enzymes, modalities, and exercise (Fig. 3-9). Two of the most interesting possibilities for treatment are the use of electrical stimulation, perhaps of low frequency, and exercise (active, resisted as opposed to stretching). Rapid intervention is important in order to restore muscular strength and power and to prevent pseudomyostatic contracture problems as well as maladaptive, compensatory movement alterations that would adversely affect the kinetic chain synergy and predispose noninvolved muscles or joints to overuse problems.

Hasson et al.[12] investigated the use of active exercise for the resolution of quadriceps DOMS with the selection of high speed (300 degrees per second), maximal effort isokinetics. The exercise was instituted 24 hours posteccentrics and the results were highly successful. In view of the extensive degree and area of damaged muscle implicated in DOMS, it is reasonable to replicate Hasson's study design with submaximal high speed movements.

Consequently, prevention of DOMS appears dependent on proper training variables and timing as well as the intrinsic process of adaptation to eccentric training, which may occur from a single bout of eccentric training with prevention of DOMS for 1 week.[25]

REFERENCES

1. Walmsley RP, Pearson N, Stymiest P: Eccentric wrist extensor contractions and the force velocity relationship in muscle. J Orthop Sports Phys Ther 8:292, 1986
2. Hardy MA: The biology of scar formation. Phys Ther 69:1017, 1989
3. Moritani T, DeVries HA: Neural factors versus hypertrophy in the time course of muscle strength gain. Am J Phys Med 58:115, 1979
4. Mannheimer JS: A comparison of strength gain between concentric and eccentric contractions. Phys Ther 49:1207, 1969
5. Johnson BL, Adamczyk JW: A Program of eccentric-concentric strength training. Am Correct Ther J 29:16, 1975
6. Knight KL: Knee rehabilitation by the daily adjustable progressive resistive exercise. Am J Sports Med 7:336, 1979
7. Curwin S, Stanish W: Tendonitis: Its Etiology and Treatment. DC Heath and Co, Lexington, KY, 1985
8. Blackburn TA: Throwing injuries to the shoulder, p. 209. In Donatelli R (ed): Physical Therapy of The Shoulder. Churchill Livingstone, New York, 1987
9. Laycoe RR, Marteniuk RG: Learning and tension as factors in static strength gains produced by static and eccentric training. Res Q 42:304, 1971
10. Duncan PW, Chandler JM, Cavanaugh DK et al: Mode and speed specificity of eccentric and concentric exercise training. J Orthop Sports Phys Ther 11:74, 1989
11. Singh M, Karpovich PV: Effect of eccentric training of agonists on antagonistic muscles. J Appl Physiol 23:744, 1967
12. Hasson S, Barnes W, Hunter M, Williams J: Thera-

peutic effect of high speed voluntary muscle contractions on muscle soreness and muscle performance. J Orthop Sports Phys Ther 10:499, 1989

13. Komi PV, Buskirk ER: Effect of eccentric and concentric muscle conditioning on tension and electrical activity of human muscle. Ergonomics 15:417, 1972
14. Griffin JW: Differences in elbow flexion torque measured concentrically, eccentrically and isometrically. Phys Ther 67:1207, 1987
15. Trudelle-Jackson E, Meske N, Highgenboten C, Jackson A: Eccentric/concentric torque deficits in the quadriceps muscle. J Orthop Sports Phys Ther 11:144, 1989
16. Fowler WM, Gardner GW, Kazerunian HH, Lauvstad WA: The effect of exercise on serum enzymes. Arch Phys Med Rehabil 49:554, 1968
17. Shumate JB, Brooke MH, Carroll JE: Increases serum CK after exercise: a sex linked phenomenon. Neurology 29:902, 1979
18. Highgenboten CL, Jackson AW, Meske NB: Concentric and eccentric torque comparisons for knee extension and flexibility in young adult males and females using the kinetic communicator. Am J Sport Med 16:236, 1988
19. Andrew P: Motor unit activity under low tensions as muscle changes length. Am J phys Med 64:248, 1985
20. Stanton P, Purdam C: Hamstring injuries in sprinting–the role of eccentric exercise. J Orthop Sports Phys Ther 10:347, 1989
21. Cote C, Simoneau JA, Lagasse P, Thibault MC, Marcotte M, Bouchard C: Isokinetic strength training protocols: do they induce skeletal muscle fiber hypertrophy? Arch Phys Med Rehabil 69:281, 1988
22. Grimby G, Gustafsson E, Peterson L, Renstrom P: Quadriceps function and training after knee ligament surgery. Med Sci Sports Exerc 12:70, 1980
23. Thomee R, Renstrom P, Grimby G, Peterson L: Slow or fast isokinetic training after surgery. J Orthop Sports Phys Ther 8:476, 1987
24. Johnson BL, Adamczyk JW, Tennoe KW, Stromme SB: A comparison of concentric and eccentric muscle training. Med Sci Sports Exer 8:35, 1976
25. Stauber WT: Eccentric action of muscles: physiology, injury and adaptation. Exerc Sports Sci Rev 19:157, 1989
26. Clarkson PM, Litchfield P, Graves J et al: Serum creatine kinase levels following forearm flexion isometric exercise. Eur J Appl Physiol 53:370, 1985
27. Clarkson PM, Byrnes WC, Gillison E, Harper E: Adaptation to exercise-induced muscle damage. Clin Sci 73:385, 1987
28. Evans WJ, Meredith CN, Cannon JG et al: Metabolic changes following eccentric exercise in trained and untrained men. J Appl Physiol 61:1865, 1986
29. Howell JN, Chila AG, Ford G et al: An electromyographic study of elbow motion during postexercise muscle soreness. J Appl Physiol 58:1713, 1985
30. Newham DJ, Clarkson PM: Repeated high-force eccentric exercise: effects on muscle pain and damage. J Appl Physiol 63:1382, 1987
31. Armstrong RB: Mechanisms of exercise-induced delayed onset muscular soreness: a brief review. Med Sci Sports Exerc 16:529, 1984
32. Byrnes WC, Clarkson PM, Katch F: Muscle soreness following resistance exercise with and without eccentric contractions. Res Q Exerc Sports 56:283, 1985
33. Chandler JM, Duncan PW: Eccentric vs. concentric force velocity relationships of the quadriceps femoris muscle, abstracted. Phys Ther 68:800, 1988
34. Nicely K, Schultz C, Porter S et al: Effects of training using isokinetic-concentric, isokinetic-eccentric and isometric contractions on the peak torque of the knee extensors, abstracted. Phys Ther 68:799, 1988
35. Ellenbecker TS, Davies GJ, Rowinski MS: Concentric versus eccentric isokinetic strengthening of the rotator cuff: objective data versus functional test. Am J Sports Med 16:64, 1988
36. Tomberlin JP, Basford JR: A comparative study of eccentric and concentric quadricep strengthening, abstracted. Phys Ther 67:790, 1987
37. Arms SW, Pope MH, Johnson RJ et al: The biomechanics of anterior curciate ligament rehabilitation and reconstruction. Am J Sports Med 12:8, 1984
38. Lieb FJ, Perry J: Quadriceps function: anatomical and mechanical study using amputated limbs. J Bone Joint Surg 50:1548, 1985
39. Olson VL. Smidt GL, Johnston RC: The maximum torque generated by the eccentric, isometric and concentric contractions of the hip abductor muscles. Phys Ther 52:156, 1972
40. Grieve GL: Common Vertebral Joint Problems. Churchill Livingstone, New York, 1981
41. Jackson CP, Brown MD: Is there a role for exercises in the treatment of patients with low back pain? Clin Orthop 179:34, 1983
42. Hood LB, Forward EM: Strength variations in two determinations of maximal isometric contractions. J Am Phys Ther 45:1046, 1965

43. Warshal D: Reliability of isometric strength gain in therapeutic assessment. Am Correct Ther J:33:188, 1979
44. Pavone E, Moffat M: Isometric torque of the quadriceps femoris after concentric, eccentric and isometric training. Arch Phys Med Rehabil 66:168, 1985
45. Newham DJ, Mills KR, Quigley BM, Edwards RHT: Pain and fatigue after concentric and eccentric muscle contractions. Clin Sci 64:55, 1983
46. Francis KT: Delayed muscle soreness: a review. J Orthop Sports Phys Ther 5:10, 1983
47. Yackzan L, Adams C. Francis KT: The effects of ice massage on delayed muscle soreness. Am J Sports Med 12:159, 1984
48. Talag TS: Residual muscular soreness as influenced by concencentric, eccentric and static contractions. Res Q 44:458, 1973
49. Byrnes WC, Clarkson PM, White JS et al: Delayed onset muscle soreness following repeated bouts of downhill running. J Appl Physiol 59:710, 1985
50. McCully KK, Faulkner JA: Injury to skeletal muscle fibers of mice following lengthening contractions. J Appl Physiol 59:119, 1985
51. Carlsson C, Pellettieri L: A clinical view on pain physiology. Acta Chir Scand 148:305, 1982
52. Clarkson PM, Tremblay I: Rapid adaptation to exercise induced muscle damage. J Appl Physiol 65:1, 1988
53. Assmussen E: Observations on experimental muscle soreness. Acta Rheumatol Scand 1:109, 1956
54. Hough T: Ergographic studies in muscular soreness. Am J Physiol 7:76, 1902
55. deVries HA: Prevention of muscular distress after exercise. Res Q 32:177, 1961
56. Eisenberg BR: Quantitative ultrastructure of mammalian skeletal muscle, p. 73. In Peachey LD, Adrian RH, Geiger SR (eds): Handbook of Physiology, Section 10, Skeletal Muscle. Waverly Press, Baltimore, 1983
57. Armstrong R, Marun P, Tullson P, Saubert C: Acute hypertrophic response of skeletal muscle to removal of synergists. J Appl Physiol 46:835, 1979
58. Garrett WE, Califf JC, Bassett FH: Histochemical correlates of hamstring injuries. Am J Sports Med 12:98, 1984
59. Friden J, Seger J, Sjostrom M, Ekblom B: Adaptive response in human skeletal muscle subjected to prolonged eccentric training. Int J Sports Med 43:177, 1983
60. Schwane J, Johnson S, Vandernakker C, Armstrong R: Blood markers of delayed-onset muscle soreness with downhill treadmill running. Med Sci Sports Exerc 13:80, 1981
61. Waltrous B, Armstrong R, Schwane J: The role of lactic acid in delayed onset muscular distress. Med Sci Sports Exerc 13:80, 1981
62. Friden J, Sjostrom M: Human muscle morphology and strength performance after long distance running. Med Sci Sports Exerc 13:81, 1981
63. Abraham WM: Factors in delayed muscle soreness. Med Sci Sports Exerc 9:11, 1977
64. Abraham WM: Exercise induced muscle soreness. Phys Sports Med 7:57, 1979
65. Armstrong RB, Ogilvie RW, Schwane JA: Eccentric exercise induced injury to rat skeletal muscle. J Appl Physiol 54:80, 1983
66. Friden J: Sublethal muscle fiber injuries after high tension anaerobic exercise. Eur J Appl Physiol 57:360, 1988
67. Friden J, Sjostrom M, Ekblom B: A morphological study of delayed muscle soreness. Experientia 37:506, 1981
68. Garrett WE, Duncan PW: Muscle injury and rehabilitation. p. 10. In Malone TR (ed): Sports Injury Management Series. Vol. 1. Williams & Wilkins, Baltimore, 1988
69. Jones DA: Muscle fatigue due to changes beyond the neuromuscular junction. p. 178. Porter R, Whelan J (eds): *Human Muscle Fatigue Physiological Mechanisms.* Ciba Symposium 82. Pitman Medical Press, London, 1981
70. Tullson PC, Armstrong RB: Exercise induced muscle inflammation. Fed Proc 37:663, 1968
71. Tullson P, Armstrong RB: Muscle hexose monophosphate shunt activity following exercise. Experientia 37:1311, 1981
72. Korvanen V, Suominen H, Heiddinen E: Mechanical properties of fast and slow skeletal muscle with special reference to collagen and endurance training. J Biomech 17:725, 1984
73. Tidball JG, Daniel TL: Elastic energy storage in rigored skeletal muscle cells under physiological loading conditions. Am J Physiol 250:R56, 1986
74. Mense S, Schmidt RF: Activation of group IV afferent units from muscle by algesic agents. Brain Res 72:305, 1974
75. Stacy MJ: Free nerve endings in skeletal muscle of the cat. J Anat 105:231, 1969
76. Carlson BM, Faulkner JA: The regeneration of skeletal muscle fibers following injury: a review. Med Sci Sports Exerc 15:187, 1983
77. Webster's Seventh New Collegiate Dictionary. G & C Merriam Co, Springfield, 1965

78. Duncan CJ: Role of calcium in triggering rapid ultrastructural damage in muscle: a study with chemically skinned fibers. J Cell Sci 87:581, 1987
79. Newham DJ: Eccentric contractions and delayed onset pain. Eur J Appl Physiol 57:372, 1988
80. Newham DJ, Jones DA, Edwards RH: Large delayed plasma creatine kinase changes after stepping exercise. Muscle Nerve 6:380, 1983
81. Vihko V, Rantamaki J, Salminen A: Exhaustive physical exercise and acid hydrolase activity in mouse skeletal muscle. Histochemistry 57:237, 1978
82. Lane RJM, Turnbull DM, Welch JL, Walton SJ: A double blind, placebo-controlled, crossover study of verapamil in exertional muscle pain. Muscle Nerve 9:635, 1986
83. Friden J, Sfakianos PN, Hargens AR: Muscle soreness and intramuscular fluid pressure: comparison between eccentric and concentric load. J Appl Physiol 61:2175, 1986
84. Wallensten R, Eklund B: Intramuscular pressures and muscle metabolism after short-term and long-term exercise. Int J Sports Med 4:231, 1983
85. Knight K: The effects of hypothermia on inflammation and swelling. Athl Train 11:7, 1976
86. Waylonis GW: The physiologic effects of ice massage. Arch Phys Med Rehabil 48:38, 1967
87. McMaster WC: A literature review on ice therapy in injuries. Am J Sports Med 5:124, 1977
88. Hill DW, Richardson JD: Effectiveness of 10% trolamine salicylate cream on muscular soreness induced by a reproducible program of weight training. J Orthop Sports Phys Ther 11:19, 1989
89. Headley S, Newham D, Jones D: The effect of prednisolone on exercise induced muscle pain and damage. Clin Sci, suppl. 13: 70:85, 1986
90. Janssen E, Kuipers H, Verstappen F, Costill D: Influence of an anti-inflammatory drug on muscle soreness. Med Sci Sports Exerc 15:165, 1983
91. Kuipers H, Keizer H, Verstappen F, Costill D: Influence of a prostaglandin inhibiting drug on muscle soreness after eccentric work. Int J Sports Med 6:336, 1985
92. Richardson RL, Denegar CO, O'Bryant HA: Contralateral and Extra segmental TENS for the relief of musculo-skeletal pain. Athl Train 24:115, 1989
93. Denegar CR, Perrin DH, Rogol AD, Rutt R: Influence of transcutaneous electrical nerve stimulation on pain, range of motion and serum cortisol concentration in females experiencing delayed onset muscle soreness. J Orthop Sports Phys Ther 11:100, 1989
94. Buroker KX, Schwane JA: Does postexercise static stretching alleviate delayed muscle soreness? Phys Sports Med 17:83, 1989
95. Clarkson PM, Byrnes WC, McCormick KM et al: Muscle soreness and serum creatine kinase activity following isometric, eccentric and concentric exercise. Int J Sports Med 3:152, 1986

4

Plyometrics

MICHAEL L. VOIGHT
PETER DRAOVITCH

Movement can be defined as a series of repeated muscular contractions regulated by neural control mechanisms that are directed by motor learning pathways. Purposeful movement is dependent upon the intimate communication of each and every muscular length and tension regulating mechanism. In athletics, success is dependent upon the speed at which these impulses are transmitted and the subsequent muscular force that is achieved. The term used to define this equation is power or work divided by time (work/time).

Power represents the one component of athletic fitness that may be most indicative of success in sports requiring extreme and rapid force production. Over the years, researchers, fitness specialists, and coaches have attempted to design strength and conditioning programs geared towards optimally activating, sensitizing, and potentially educating this force production system. Power can be increased by either increasing the amount of work or force that is produced by the muscles or by decreasing the amount of time required to produce the force. The overload principle provides the athlete with a means of improving strength levels. Practice of skill pattern components increases the speed and efficiency of practiced movement patterns. The amount of time required to produce muscular force is the important variable for increased power. One form of training that theoretically proposes to bridge the gap between speed and strength is plyometrics.[1]

The term *plyometrics* was introduced into the United States by track and field coach Fred Wilt.[2] The origin of the term is unknown. "Plyo" comes from the Greek word "pleythein," which means to increase. "Plyo" is the Greek word for "more," while "metric" means to measure. Despite the unclear history, the term plyometrics is relatively new; however, the concept is old. Many believe that the Eastern block countries were the originators of plyometric training following their performance in the 1972 Olympics. Articles were published in athletic magazines detailing a strange system of jumps and bounds that were utilized by the Soviets to increase speed. It was discovered that the concept of plyometrics was not new. American coaches had been utilizing forms of plyometric training such as bench hops and rope jumping for many years without understanding the concept. What the Eastern block sport scientists did master was the organization of the concept. This has been credited to the legendary Soviet jump coach Yuri Verhoshanski.[3]

The practical definition of plyometrics is a quick powerful movement involving a prestretching or countermovement that activates the stretch shortening cycle. The purpose of plyometric training is to heighten the excitability of the nervous system for improved reactive ability of the neuromuscular system. Any exercise that utilizes the natural elastic components of muscle and the myotatic reflex to produce a more powerful muscular response is plyometric in nature. Because all movement in both competitive athletics and normal activities of daily living (ADL) involves a repeated series of stretch shortening cycles, specific functional exercise must be used to prepare the individual for their activity utilizing plyometric training.

Quickness in movement is a key factor in athletic performance. The less time spent on the ground in one place is of paramount importance. Vermiel[4] developed a formula to assess ground reaction time. The efficiency is the relationship between the time spent on the ground and the vertical height achieved during jumping. The goal of plyometric training is the reduction of the amortization time phase. This phase is the amount of time between undergoing a yielding eccentric phase and initiating an overcoming concentric contraction.

This chapter will attempt to familiarize the reader with the physiologic principles on which plyometrics are based. In addition, practical applications based on these principles will be discussed for specific sports and populations, including children. Clinical applications for rehabilitating patients will also be addressed. Finally, examples of program design, equipment utilization, and the basis for incorporating plyometric into the overall strength and conditioning rehabilitation program will be provided.

PHYSIOLOGIC PRINCIPLES

Traditional muscle physiology has in the past focused on both the motor and stabilization action of the muscular system; however, the important action of shock absorption or spring-like action cannot be forgotten. Motor function centers around muscle contractions that involve muscle shortening, during which the muscle system attempts to overcome an external force. If the external force overcomes the muscle ability to actively resist, the muscle lengthens. This lengthening occurs only after additional force is produced. In normal function, muscle action seldom begins from a static starting position. In most activities the muscle is stretched before it contracts concentrically. This eccentric-concentric coupling is also referred to as the *stretch shortening cycle*. The physiology of a muscular response is usually attributed to the inherent proprioceptive reflexes and the elastic characteristics of the muscle undergoing contraction. For the purpose of explanation and understanding, the elastic mechanical characteristics and reflexive properties of the muscular system will be discussed separately, although they function simultaneously.

Muscle behavior is often represented as a three-component model (Fig. 4-1). Within this model the three mechanical characteristics of muscle can be demonstrated. A contractile component (CC), series elastic component (SEC), and parallel elastic component (PEC) all play important roles in the generation of force. While the CC is easily understood, the SEC and PEC symbolize different structures that can act like springs and either lengthen or stretch. The behavior of an actively contracting muscle is represented by the CC and SEC. With concentric muscle contraction some stretching of the SEC occurs; however, most of the force is produced by the muscle fiber filaments' sliding past one another. The CC generates the force that is registered externally by being transferred through the SEC (Fig. 4-2). When eccentric contraction occurs, the muscle lengthens like a spring as it contracts. With this lengthening the SEC is also stretched and allowed to contribute to the force production. Therefore, the total force produced is the sum of that produced by the CC and the stretching of the SEC (Fig. 4-3).

Several authors have shown that an eccentric contraction immediately preceding a concentric contraction will significantly increase the force generated concentrically due to the storage of

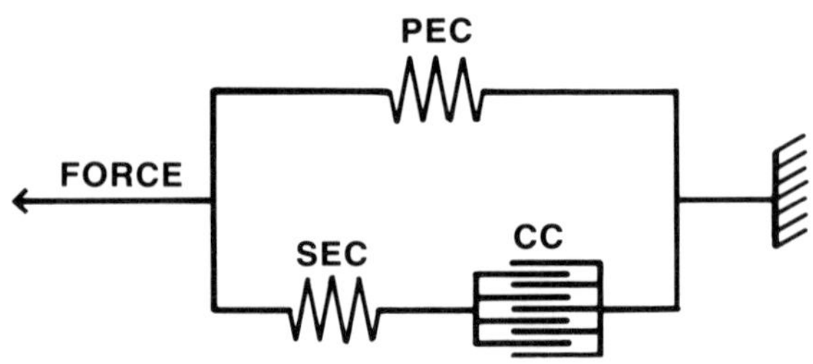

Fig. 4-1. Three-component model of muscle behavior. PEC, parallel plastic component; SEC, series elastic component; CC, contractile component.

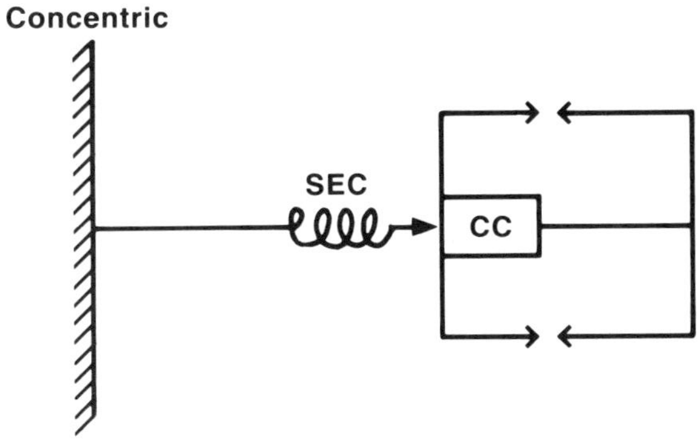

Fig. 4-2. Muscle behavior—concentric contraction. SEC, series elastics component; CC, contractile component.

elastic energy.[5–7] The mechanism for this increase in concentric force is the ability of the muscle to utilize the force produced by the SEC. During eccentric contraction the load is transferred to the SEC and stored as elastic energy. As the muscle undergoes concentric contraction, the elastic energy stored in the SEC can be recovered and used to contribute to the shortening contraction. The ability to use stored elastic energy is affected by three variables: time, magnitude of stretch, and velocity of stretch.[8] Enhancement of the concentric contraction is most effective when the preceding eccentric contraction is of short range and performed quickly without delay.[5–7] This quick change in direction is the important factor when utilizing the elastic components of the muscle.

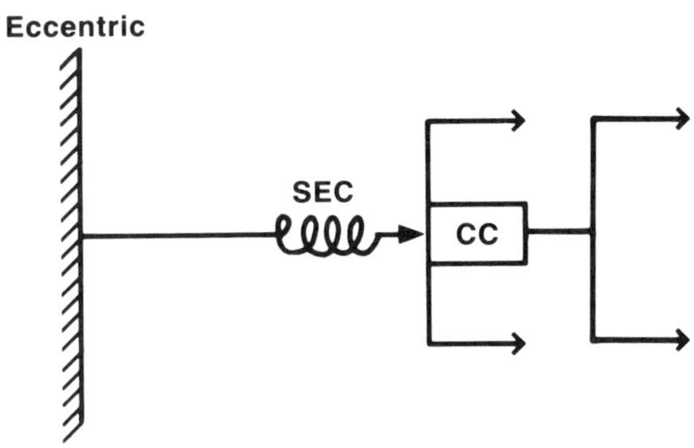

Fig. 4-3. Muscle behavior—eccentric contraction. SEC, series elastic component; CC, contractile component.

Bosco and Komi[6] demonstrated this experimentally when they compared "damped" and "undamped" depth jumps. In an undamped landing from a depth jump, there was minimal flexion at the knee with a rebound jump. Damped landings included an increase in knee flexion and time prior to the corresponding rebound jump. The investigators concluded that the power values were much higher for the undamped versus the damped groups due to the fact that the elasticity of the muscles decreased as knee flexion increased. The increased flexion at the knees during the damped jumps affected the short range stiffness of the muscle thereby causing part of the elastic energy to be dissipated as heat.

The proprioceptive stretch reflex is another positive force producing mechanism that is related to the behavior of muscle during the stretch shortening cycle. Musculoskeletal motor control is regulated by the central nervous system (CNS). Proprioceptors located within the muscle provide afferent information about the degree of muscular distortion. This information is then capable of influencing muscle tone, motor execution programs, and kinesthetic awareness. The proprioceptors of prime concern in understanding the neurophysiology of plyometrics are the Golgi tendon organs (GTO) and muscle spindles.[9]

The muscle spindle, a small complex organ located within the muscle fibers, has both afferent and efferent innervation. It functions mainly as a stretch receptor. Sensory information is transmitted to the CNS via afferent axons that inform the other neurons in the spinal cord and brain of the length of the muscle spindle and the rate at which it is being stretched. The muscle spindle also contains contractile fibers that are controlled by small gamma efferents from the spinal cord. If the length of the surrounding muscle fibers is less than that of the spindle, the frequency of nerve impulses discharged from the receptors is reduced. When the muscle spindle is activated via stretching, a sensory afferent response is evoked and transmitted to the spinal cord, which in turn sends impulses back to the muscle causing a motor response (Fig. 4-4). Shortening of the muscle relieves the stretch on the muscle spindles contained within the muscle, thereby removing

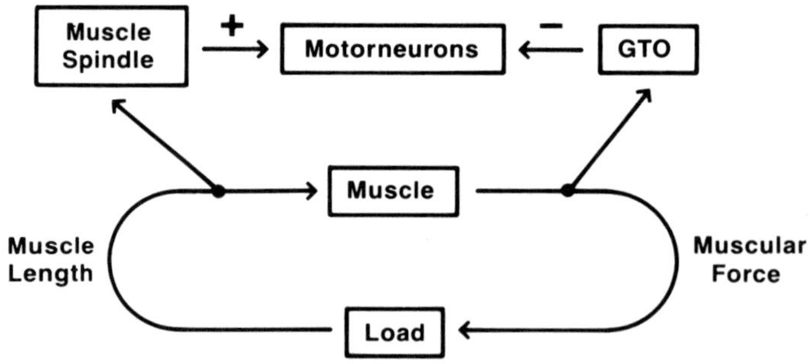

Fig. 4-4. Neuromuscular response loops. GTO, Golgi tendon organs.

the stimulus from the stretch receptors. This process is called the stretch or myotatic reflex. This is the only monosynaptic reflex in the body. The loop time for the stretch reflex is between 30 to 50 milliseconds, while additional reflex loop times are available by consulting Table 4-1. The strength of the muscle spindles response to stretch is determined by the rate of stretch.[9] The greater and more quickly a load is applied to a muscle, the greater the firing frequency of the muscle spindle with a corresponding stronger muscle contraction.

Golgi tendon organs that lie within muscle tendons near the point of attachment of the muscle fiber to the tendon are involved in a tension limiting reflex. Unlike the muscle spindle, the GTO has an inhibitory effect on the muscle. Due to the GTOs series alignment with the contractile muscle fibers, activation occurs with stretch. When deformation or tension is produced, sensory impulses are transmitted rapidly to the spinal cord and the cerebellum. The arrival of these impulses at the spinal cord causes inhibition of the alpha motor neurons of the contracting muscle and its synergists thereby limiting the force developed.

During a muscle contraction, the activity from the muscle spindle is reduced because the muscle fibers are either shortening or attempting to shorten. During an eccentric contraction, the muscle stretch reflex acts to generate more tension in the lengthening muscle. When the muscle tension increases to a high or potentially harmful level, the GTO fires thereby generating a neural pattern that reduces the excitation of the muscle. While the GTO fires in response to high muscular tension or stretch, the inhibitory effect may be offset

Table 4-1. Four Kinds of Responses to Environmental Stimuli During Movement, and Some of Their Differing Characteristics

		Category of Analysis		
Response Type	Loop Time (msec)	Structures Involved	Modified by Instructions	Affected by No. of Choices
Myotatic reflexes (autogenetic)	30–50	Spindles, gamma loop, same muscles	No	No
Long-loop reflexes (autogenetic)	50–80	Spindles, cortex or cerebellum, same muscles	Yes	No
Triggered reactions (not autogenetic)	80–120	Various receptors, higher centers, and associated musculature	Yes	Yes
Reaction time (not autogenetic)	120–180	Various receptors, higher centers, any musculature	Yes	Yes

(From Schmidt,[53] with permission.)

during voluntary exertion until the muscular tension becomes excessive and the potential for injury is increased.

As these two systems oppose each other, increased muscular force is produced. The descending pathways from the brain must balance these forces and ultimately control which reflex will dominate.[10]

Improvement in skeletal muscle performance that occurs with initial prestretching of the muscle can be identified as the combined effects of both the storage of elastic energy and the myotatic reflex activation of the muscle.[5,6,7,11–13] The percentage of contribution from each component is not known at this time.[6] The degree of improvement is dependent upon the time frame between the eccentric and subsequent concentric contractions.[7] This time frame can be defined as the amortization phase.[1] The amortization phase can best be defined as the electromechanical delay between eccentric and concentric contraction during which the muscle must switch from overcoming work to imparting the necessary amount of acceleration in the required direction.

One study that compared men and women found that although men created more tension, women were better able to use stored elastic energy.[14] Komi[15] reports that the greatest tension developed during the stretch-shortening cycle occurs during muscle lengthening just prior to the concentric contraction. He concludes that the increase in the amortization phase causes a decrease in muscle tension. Stauber[16] also points out that the stretch-shortening cycle may be quite different from the eccentric contraction that occurs during shock absorption.

Plyometric training may improve physiologic performance in several ways. Training to increase the speed of the stretch reflex has not been documented; however, it has been speculated that the intensity of the subsequent muscular contraction can be increased through better recruitment of additional motor units.[17] It has been well documented in the literature that the faster a muscle is eccentrically loaded or lengthened, the greater the resultant concentric force produced. Eccentric lengthening also loads the elastic components of the muscular system and thereby the tension of the resultant rebound force. The stretch reflex may increase the stiffness of the muscular spring by recruiting additional muscle fibers that would not be possible with concentric contraction.[17] The additional stiffness may allow the muscular system to reutilize more of the external stress in the form of elastic recoil.[17] The question of improving the speed of the myotatic reflex loop still remains.

Another possible mechanism for increased force or power production with plyometic training involves the inhibitory effect of GTOs on force production. Since the GTO serves as a protective mechanism limiting the amount of force produced within a muscle, its stimulation threshold becomes the limiting factor. Bosco and Komi[6] have suggested that with stressful explosive training the GTO may become desensitized thereby raising the level of inhibition and ultimately allowing increased force production in greater loads applied to the musculoskeletal system.

The final possible mechanism in which plyometric training improves muscular performance centers around neuromuscular coordination. The speed of exertion may be limited by neuromuscular coordination. This means that the body will only move within a range of speed set by the nervous system no matter how strong the muscle system is. Training with an explosive prestretch improves neural efficiency and thereby increases neuromuscular performance. Plyometrics may cause changes within the nervous system that allow an individual to better coordinate the activities of the muscle groups thereby affecting a greater net force even in the absence of morphologic adaption within the muscles themselves. The possible changes within the nervous system that enhance strength and power performance may be referred to as a neural adaption. The nervous system may be enhanced to become more autonomic.

In conclusion, successful plyometric training relies more on the rate of stretch rather than the length of the stretch. Also, if the amortization phase is slow, elastic energy is wasted as heat and the stretch reflex is not activated. However, the more quickly the athlete is able to switch from yielding work to overcoming work, then the more powerful the response. Future understanding and success of plyometric training is dependent upon communication and mutual feedback between scientists and coaches.

PROGRAM DEVELOPMENT

Program development begins by establishing an adequate strength base. The body must be prepared to withstand the stress of plyometric training. The goal of developing a greater strength base is muscle hypertrophy that ultimately results in greater force via an increased cross-sectional area. A larger cross-sectional area can also contribute to the SEC and therefore more stored elastic energy.

While strength is commonly associated with morphologic changes within the muscle, neural mechanisms and motor learning pathways play equally important roles for the initial and quite possibly later stage gains seen in strength training.[18–22] Changes in connective tissue strength can be achieved in one of two fashions, either low repetition, high intensity load bearing or low intensity training at high volumes of repetitions. This will provide the required overload to produce accommodating strength gains. In order to realize optimal strength gains, a structured plan must be instituted to prevent potential over-use injuries.

Hortobagyi and Matveyev[23,24] divided the training schedule into the preparation period, competition period, and the first and second transition periods. Plyometric training must parallel the other incorporated components of the athlete's training schedule to prevent overtraining.[25] In order to prevent overtraining but ensure that maximum strength gains are realized, planning the training schedule should include long-term goals. These goals are influenced by factors such as when to increase the training loads, how to modify the periodization, and when to modify the composition of training.[23]

Plyometric exercises can be characterized as rapid eccentric loading of the musculoskeletal complex.[17] Plyometrics serve to train the neuromuscular system by teaching it to better accept the increased strength loads.[25] Exploitation of the stretch reflex improves the ability of the nervous system to react with maximal speed to the lengthening muscle, thereby inceasing the ability of the muscle to concentrically shorten with maximal force. Since plyometric training attempts to model the neuromuscular system, plyometric programs should be designed keeping sport specificity in mind.[26] Simply stated, all programs should be designed to incorporate the specific adaptation to imposed demands (SAID) principle.[27] This will ensure that the body is prepared to accept the stresses that will be imparted upon it in its respective athletic environment.

Matveyev's model of periodization (Fig. 4-5) employs the modification of two training variables, volume and intensity. Success of the plyometric program is based on how well the supervisor is able to control, modify, and manipulate these two variables:

1. As intensity increases, volume decreases.
2. As volume increases, intensity decreases.

Therefore, although the principle appears simple, the task of regulating this concept is sometimes difficult. The key to successfully controlling these variables is to be flexible and to listen to what the athlete's body is telling you. The athlete's body response will dictate the speed at which you are able to progress the program. When in doubt about the amount of plyometric work to be performed, it is much better to underprescribe the volume in order to prevent overuse injuries.

In order to minimize the risks for potential injury, a thorough medical history, structural evaluation, and functional testing should be performed. This will help the practitioner to determine if any prior or existing medical or orthopaedic condition would warrant disqualification from participation.[17] Once the patient has been cleared to participate in a plyometric program, the precautionary tips listed in Table 4-2 should be followed to ensure the safety of each athlete.[25,28]

While plyometrics are demanding and place considerable stress on the body, when introduced

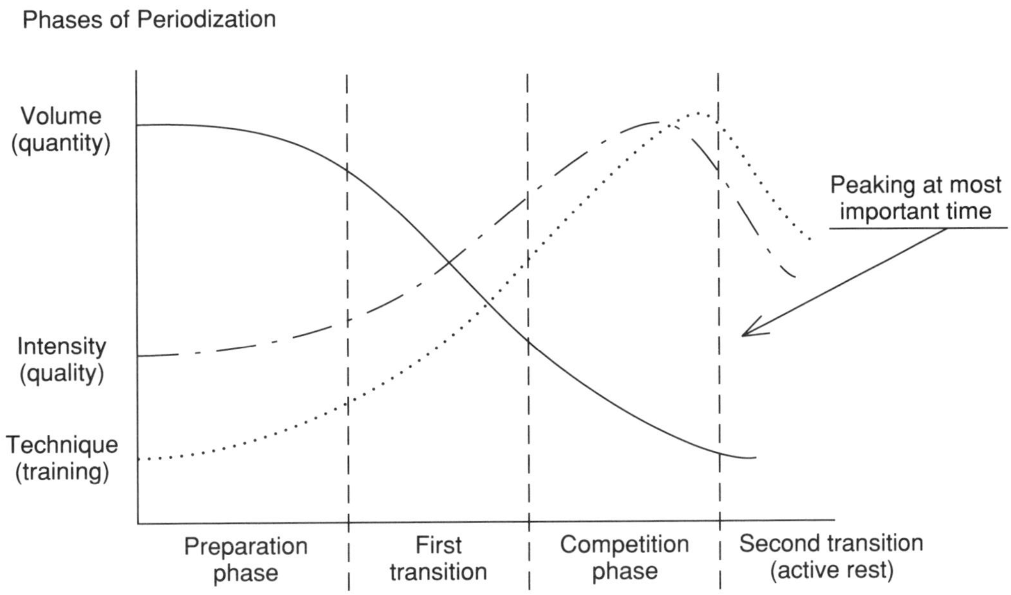

Fig. 4-5. Matveyev's model of periodization. (From Plyometric Training,[54] with permission. Copyright NSCA 1988.)

Table 4-2. Safety Requirements for Plyometric Training

Never begin a plyometric training program before a medical and orthopedic screening examination has been conducted.

Make sure that the participant has reached a basic maturation level.

Develop an adequate strength base.

Always use good supportive shoes.

Always use a good resilient surface.

Always warmup and prestretch.

Always use a progressive overload (SAID principle)

Always utilize a proper organized progression.

Make sure the participant can demonstrate proper landing before rebounding is taught.

Never accept mediocrity with technique.

Always train with knowledgable supervision.

In addition to these general safety considerations, the instructor should look at several special considerations when developing the plyometric progression:

What is the participant's body structure?

What is the participant's body size?

What is the participant's injury history?

What role will fatigue play in the program?

slowly into the conditioning program they can be safe. The Eastern block countries have arbitrarily selected a one repetition maximum in the squat at 1.5 to 2 times the person's body weight, before lower body plyometrics may be initiated.[25] Chu[1,17,29] has divided the lower extremity plyometrics into six categories: in-place jumps, standing jumps, multiple response hops and jumps, in-depth jumps and box drills, bounding, and high stress sport specific plyometrics. The National Strength and Conditioning Association classifies plyometric training as in-place, short response, and long response. The volume and intensity of plyometric training within each of these catagories can be regulated from low to high stress, thereby creating a stress continuum (Table 4-3). When the individual can demonstrate both static and dynamic control of their own body weight with single leg squats, low intensity in-place plyometrics can be initiated.

Preplyometric testing can be divided into two subcatagories, static stability and dynamic movement testing. The purpose of static stability testing is to determine the individual's ability to stabilize the torso and control the body. It is extremely

Table 4-3. Plyometric Stress Continuum

	Low (Beginner)	Medium (Intermediate)	High (Advanced)	Shock
In-place	Angle bounce Tuck jump Split jump Lateral bounce Ice skater Spin jump Lateral cone jump	Cycle jump Drop jump Jump up Lateral hop	Hops	In-depth jump[a]
Short response (≤10)	Standing long jump[a]	Three continuous standing long jumps[a] Standing triple jump[a] Single hurdle jump Skis Zig zag bounds Crossover lateral bounds 5 + hops[a] 5 + bounds[a]	Five continuous standing long jumps[a] Double-leg box jump 5–10 Hurdle rebound jumps Lateral hop 5 + hops	Continuous hurdle hops Box bounds
Long response (≥10)	Leaps	10 + bounds	10 + hops Hop/step Speed bounds	
Upper body	2-hand overhead forward throw Chest pass Half twist and full twist Walking twist with lunge Clap pushups Medicine ball pushups	Overhead backward throw in place[a] Overhead backward throw with 2 jumps[a] Underhand forward throw in place[a] Underhand forward throw with 2 jumps[a] Russian twist Drop pushups	Drop rebound pushups	1-arm pushups

[a] Suitable for testing purposes.
(From Plyometric Training,[54] with permission. Copyright NSCA 1988.)

important that the muscles of postural support are strong enough to withstand the stress of explosive training. The weaker areas of the body are often sites of injury in training. In many cases, the larger stronger muscles will cover up or hide weakness in the smaller stabilizing muscles. If a weakness is discovered, limitation within the individual's program and specific isolated strengthening exercises can be initiated.

With static testing, there are several guidelines

that the tester must bear in mind prior to the initiation of the test:

1. Each test position is held for 30 seconds.
2. The individual should be observed for shaking or "wobbling" of the extremity joints. If there is more movement of a weight-bearing joint in one direction than the other, the musculature producing movement in the opposite direction needs to be assessed for specific weakness.
3. The specific testing surface should be consistent. Any surface will suffice for testing; however, a hard surface is preferable due to its stability and consistency. Testing the individual on a soft surface will provide an overload in the stability test. The key to testing is reproducibility.
4. The individual should maintain proper upright postural alignment during testing.
5. Performance of static testing in front of a mirror may provide important feedback to the individual regarding body position.

Static stability testing (Table 4-4 and Fig. 4-6) begins with simple movements of low motor complexity and progresses to more difficult high motor skills. The basis for lower quarter stability testing centers around single leg stance. Difficulty can be increased by having the individual being tested close his or her eyes. The three basic static tests are one-legged standing, single-leg quarter squats, and single-leg half squats. An individual should be able to perform one-legged standing for 30 seconds with eyes opened and closed prior to the initiation of a plyometric program. For dynamic jump exercises to be initiated, there should be no "wobbling" of the support leg in quarter knee squats. Half squatting is a more difficult skill and should be used to assess the effectiveness of the training program.

Table 4-4. Plyometric Static Stability Testing

Single leg stance - 30 s
Eyes open
Eyes closed
Single leg quarter squat - 30 s
Eyes open
Eyes closed
Single leg half squat - 30 s
Eyes open
Eyes closed

Dynamic movement testing assesses the individual's ability to produce explosive coordinated movement. Vertical jumping for the lower quarter and medicine ball toss for the upper quarter are used to assess progress.

Before plyometric training can be initiated, the athlete and instructor must be made aware of some general guidelines. These guidelines must be strictly adhered to as any deviation away from the designed functional progression will result in minimal improvement and risk of injury. The general guidelines that must be considered before embarking on a plyometric program include the following:

1. Plyometric training should be specific to the goals established for the athlete. If the goal is to improve vertical jump, jumping would be the best method of training. Since jumping is a complex motor skill requiring coordinated movement of the body, the only way to simulate jumping is to jump. Activity specific movement patterns should be trained. The instructor should try to simulate the specific motions that are inherent to the individual's sport or activity.
2. Sport-specific skills should be broken down and trained in their smaller components and then rebuilt into a coordinated movement pattern.
3. The quality of work is more important than the quantity of work. Exercise intensity should be at a maximal level. Training at a level that is less than 100 percent will be of minimal value.
4. The greater the amplitude or intensity, the greater the recovery time.
5. Plyometric training may have its greatest benefit at the conclusion of the normal workout or practice session. This will best replicate exercise under a partial to total fatigue environment that is specific to activity. It is recommended that only low to medium stress plyometrics be used at the conclusion of a

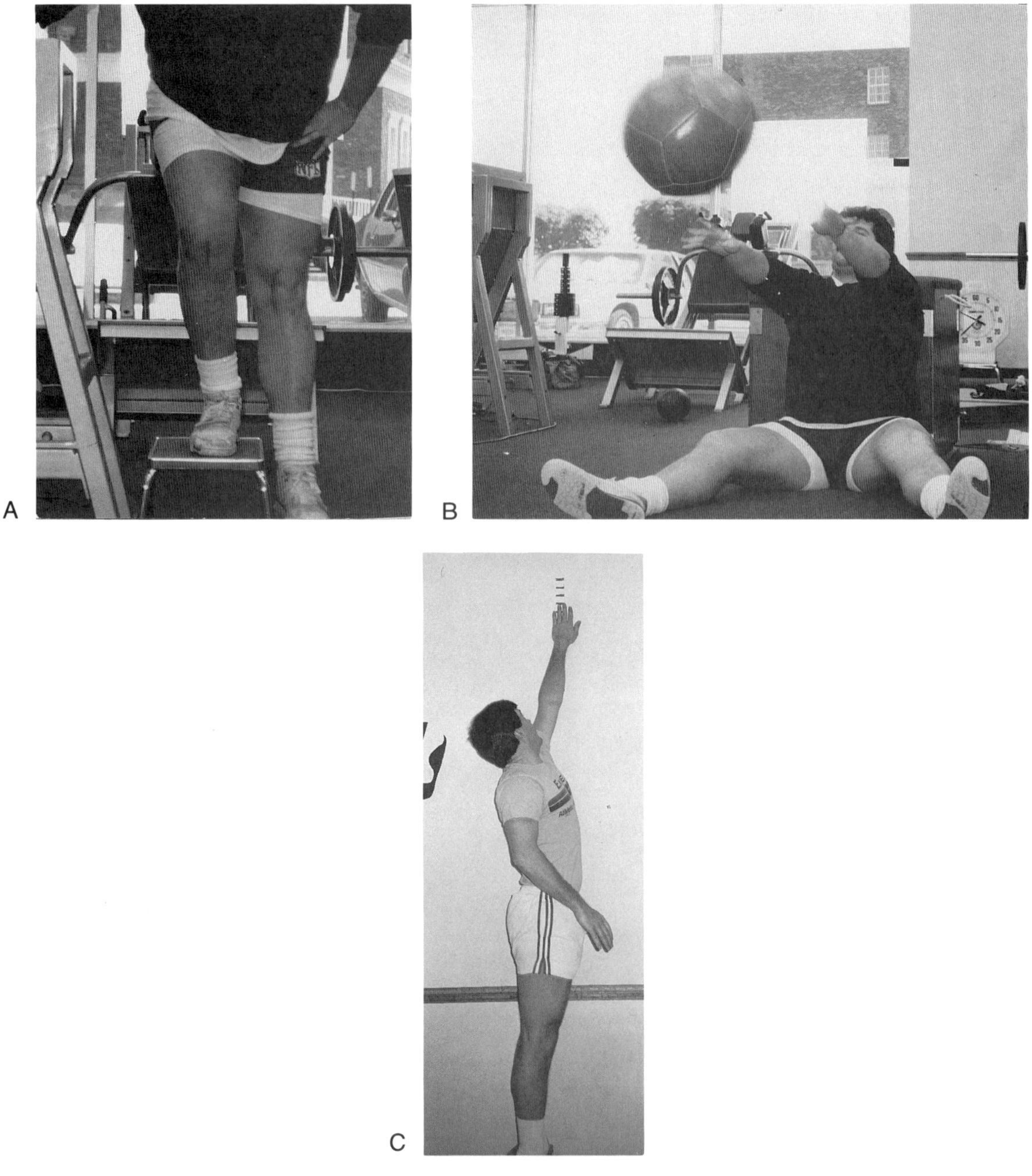

Fig. 4-6. Static stability and dynamic movement testing. Such testing is necessary to establish commencement of exercises and baseline for assessing progress. **(A)** Single leg squat as a static stability test. **(B)** Medicine ball toss. **(C)** Vertical jump. Figs. B and C measure upper quarter and lower quarter power, respectively.

workout due to the potential of injury with high stress or shock method plyometrics.

6. When the proper technique can no longer be demonstrated, maximum volume has been achieved and the exercise must be stopped.
7. In the preparatory phase, exercises of low motor complexity and intensity should dominate.
8. In the competitive phase, exercises of higher motor complexity and intensity should dominate.
9. Plyometric training sessions should be conducted no more than three times weekly during the preparatory phase and two times weekly during the competitive period.
10. Volume will prevail in the preparatory period with intensity becoming more important during the competitive period.
11. The plyometric training program should be progressive in overload. The volume and intensity can be manipulated in several ways:
    A. Increase the number of exercises.
    B. Increase the number of repetitions and sets.
    C. Change the surface or exercise equipment used.
    D. Decrease the rest period between sets or exercises.
12. Dynamic testing of the individual on a regular basis will provide important motivational feedback as well as feedback as to the progress of the plyometric program.

Table 4-5. Comprehensive Program I (Example)

Monday
- Moderate to high intensity plyometric workout
- Total body stretching program
- Skill development session
- Abdominal/low back body weight progression

Tuesday
- Moderate weight training routine (upper/lower body)
- Total body stretching program
- High intensity/low volume running program
- Abdominal/low back body weight progression

Wednesday
- Fartlek training low intensity running program
- Skill development session
- Submaximal pullup/dip routine
- Total body stretching program

Thursday
- Off

Friday
- Low intensity plyometric warmup
- Heavy weight training routine (upper/lower body)
- Total body stretching program
- Abdominal/low back weight progression

Saturday
- Moderate intensity/moderate volume running program
- Total body stretching program
- Skill development session
- Abdominal/low back body weight progression

Sunday
- Off

Program was designed in collaboration with Bill Foran, Head Strength and Conditioning Coach of the NBA's Miami Heat.

Table 4-6. Comprehensive Program II (Example)

Monday
- Moderate-high intensity plyometric workout
- Total body stretching program
- Skill development session

Tuesday
- Heavy pushing movement weight training routine
- Moderate intensity/low volume running program
- Total body stretching program
- Abdominal/low back body weight progression

Wednesday
- Heavy pulling movement/leg weight training routine
- Total body stretching program
- Skill development session
- Abdominal/low back body weight progression

Thursday
- Low intensity plyometric warmup
- Low intensity fartlek training program
- Total body stretching program

Friday
- Moderate-heavy pushing movement weight training routine
- Total body stretching program
- Skill development session
- Abdominal/low back body weight progression

Saturday
- Moderate-heavy pulling movement/leg weight training routine
- High intensity/low volume running program
- Total body stretching program
- Abdominal/low back body weight progression

Sunday
- Off

Program was designed for well conditioned, elite-level athletes. Therefore, discretion and modifications are necessary for anyone not considered to categorically represent this group. Program was designed in collaboration with Bill Foran, Head Strength and Conditioning Coach of the NBA's Miami Heat.

Table 4-7. Exercise Emphasis (Conditioning)

Phase	Duration	Volume/Intensity	Jumps/Throws
Onset	4–6 weeks	High/low	50–150/50–100
General	8 weeks	Moderate/low-moderate	100–120/50–150
Specific	6 weeks	Moderate/moderate-high	100–150/50–150
Peak	4 weeks	Low/moderate-high	80–120/50–100
In-season	Scheduled	Low/moderate-high	50–100/50–60

(From Chu,[55] with permission.)

Table 4-8. Plyometric Program (Anaerobic Sports)

Component Breakdown (%)	Frequency	Rest
Weight training (40)	2–3 days/week	2–3 days
Plyometrics (35)		
Running program (25)		

(From Chu,[55] with permission.)

Since the key to plyometrics is to maximize the force by minimizing the time, an appreciable amount of stress is placed on the musculoskeletal system. The most important prerequisite for plyometric training is the development of general and specific flexibility. Therefore, a plyometric program should include a general warm-up and cool down, as well as mandatory pre- and post-workout flexibility exercises. The warm-up should produce mild sweating,[30] whereas the flexibility exercises should be both static and short dynamic in nature.[28] The plyometric workout should be individualized, progressive, and sport specific[30,31] (Tables 4-5 to 4-9). The monitoring of the plyometric routines is essential for two reasons. First, immediate appropriate feedback is available for the athlete regarding proper techniques. Second, signs of fatigue and overtraining can be observed and the workout can be terminated. Some of the more common signs of fatigue and overtraining are noted in Table 4-10.[24,25]

Rest periods should be from 1 to 2 minutes for low intensity exercises and 3 to 5 minutes for high intensity exercises. If greater rest time is needed it should be done actively. It is recommended that the rest period between exercise sessions should be 3 to 4 days.

Table 4-9. Plyometric Workout Example (General Conditioning Phase)

1. Warmup 10–20 min
2. Low intensity jump drills, 3–5 exercises, 10–20 repetitions
3. Moderate intensity jump drills, 3–4 exercises, 5–8 repetitions
4. High intensity jump drills, 2–3 exercises, 10–20 repetitions
5. Medicine ball drills, 100 throws

(From Chu,[55] with permission.)

CHILDREN AND PLYOMETRICS

Today, it is estimated that there are more than 20 million children and adolescents participating in organized sports.[32] Of that 20 million, more than

Table 4-10. Signs of Fatigue and Overtraining

Prolonged foot contact
Excessive body lead
Lack of arm/leg coordination
Reduced vertical height and horizontal distance
Longer rest periods
Lack of synchronous head and trunk movement
Loss of interest

7 million are involved in scholastic programs.[33] Many physiologic and psychological differences exist between these young athletes and their adult counterparts. Since the emphasis by society has been on winning, preparation for success continues to begin at an earlier age. Before a training program is developed, all avenues must be explored regarding the adaptations of training on specific body systems.[34] The program should be designed to develop motor skills, but there is controversy regarding the use of weight training and its effect on the skeletally immature athlete. Since an adequate strength base is a requirement for participation in a plyometric program, it is essential that this topic be thoroughly reviewed. Opponents of weight training contend that sufficient amounts of circulating androgens are not present; resistance training would therefore be dangerous and gains would not improve performance or reduce injury at this level.[35] Currently, research demonstrates that prepubescent children involved in weight training programs can improve strength levels without causing damage to the musculoskeletal structures.[36] It should be emphasized however, that the program be strictly supervised by expert professionals stressing low resistance with a higher number of repetitions.[37]

Because of an immature CNS and low threshold GTO, children may not tolerate excessive eccentric loads produced by plyometric training.[25,38] This may serve as a natural protective mechanism by the body against excessive forces. According to the president of the National Association of Speed and Explosion, plyometrics are not recommended for children. The rapid exposure of plyometics has lead to its increased popularity; however, research is lacking.[39]

Before any new training technique is incorporated into the program, serious considerations should be given to the potential for injury that accompanies that new training method.[40] Children at the greatest risk for injury are those currently undergoing a growth spurt, especially those in Tanner stage III of development. Tanner stage III represents the stage of growth when the maximum spurt of vertical height is achieved. During this stage the growth plate is most vulnerable to injury.[33] In the growing skeleton, growth cartilage can be found at the epiphyseal plate, the joint surface, and the apophyseal insertion.[41] Because of the extreme force production that accompanies plyometric training, the growth spurt during Tanner stage III of development should serve as a major indicator for modifying the periodized plyometric program. Flexibility exercises should be the number one priority in the athlete undergoing a growth spurt. Stanitski[33] advocates the six "S's" rule in the prevention or management of stress injuries. The six S's are shoes, surface, speed, structure, strength, and stretching. Speed is the one factor most often implicated in overuse injuries. This is commonly referred to as "too much, too soon." The safety requirements for plyometric training very much resemble the six factors presented by Bielik et al.[25] and Stanitski.[33] Therefore, prevention of overuse injuries is possible if the safety requirements are strictly adhered to and the growth factor is allowed to dictate the volume and intensity of the program.

Children at play are repeatedly exposed to plyometric type exercises throughout the day. Examples of this include hop scotch, jumping rope, dodge ball, and assorted relay races. Emphasis should be placed on teaching proper technique. Proper technique should include full foot landings; the necessity of spending as little time as possible on the ground should be stressed. Prerequisites for beginning a child's program are as follows:

1. Pushups (5)
2. Squat thrusts (5)
3. Standing long jumps (athlete's height)
4. Jumping rope (30 seconds)
5. Square patterns—jumps and hops

Once a child has been able to demonstrate the above mentioned skills, his initial program should consist of low intensity in-place plyometic drills (Table 4-3).

In conclusion, societal acceptance of coeducational competitive youth sports programs could invite increased training intensity among young athletes. Potential physiologic limits of these young athletes remain relatively unexplored. The effects of plyometrics on growing children are un-

Table 4-11. Plyometrics for Children

1. Require a medical and structural clearing examination.
2. Provide knowledgeable supervision.
3. Demand proper technique and execution.
4. Allow growth and maturation patterns to dictate volume and intensity of the program.
5. Institute a policy that requires re-evaluation and clearance before progressing to the next level of plyometrics.
6. Modify the program as physical or psychological insult dictates.
7. Avoid high intensity and shock level activities while using discretion with medium intensity skills.
8. Emphasize a daily total body flexibility program.
9. Design the program utilizing play.
10. Discontinue plyometrics if it appears that the participant is no longer having fun.

known while the structural abnormalities, commonly seen in growing girls, require further discussion. The inability of children to tolerate high eccentric loads causes even more confusion about the efficacy of plyometric training for children. However, it would be unrealistic to believe that children are not exposed to forces during play that are equal to and probably exceed those forces that would have to be tolerated during a low intensity in-place plyometric program. Table 4-11 provides suggestions to ensure that a safe but effective program will be designed, implemented, and followed.

LOWER QUARTER TRAINING

Initiation of a lower quarter plyometric program first begins with low intensity in-place and multiple response jumping. Intensity is progressively increased to high intensity stress/shock training with depth jumps (Table 4-3). Depth jumping was first described by Verhoshanski and Chornonson[3] and Verhoshanski[42] when they published specific heights for 1- and 2-foot drop landings. They described the depth jump as a straight line drop from a height of .75 and 1.10 meters. This form of plyometric exercise requires that the athlete step off a box and upon making contact with the ground, move the body directly upward as rapidly as possibly.[17] The athlete is instructed to "touch and go." The analogy of jumping onto a hot bed of coals is often used to emphasize the point of quick rebounding.

Since the main concern in plyometric training is the intensity of contraction and the rate at which the resultant stretch-reflex response occurs, performing depth jumps from boxes of varying heights can be a great value. There has been a lack of agreement among researchers as to the optimum height for depth jumping. Clinically, lower box heights are used for children and untrained individuals while more experienced and higher trained athletes use higher box heights. Verhoshanski and Chornonson[3] concluded that dropping from a height greater than 42 inches is counter-

Table 4-12. Depth Jump and Trunk Progressions

Depth jump progression
- Box drop—rebound for maximal height
- Box drop—rebound linear for distance
- Box drop—rebound to another box
- Box drop—rebound vertically, sprint upon landing
- Box drop—rebound linearly, sprint upon landing
- Repeat above sequence with one leg hops
- Repeat entire sequence with light-weight vest or hand weights

Trunk progression
- Partner medicine ball
    - Seated/standing rotations
    - Seated/standing Figure 8s
- Weight plate
    - Sunrise/sunset
    - Rotations (Russian twist)
    - Revolutions (CW/CCW)
    - Figure 8s
    - Diagonals

Situp program
- Pelvic tilts
- Crunches
    - Legs supported
    - Legs unsupported
    - With twist
- Diver (pike) situps
- Medicine ball situps
    - Chest
    - Overhead
    - Right/left
- Medicine ball incline situps

Abbreviations: CW, clockwise; CCW, counterclockwise.

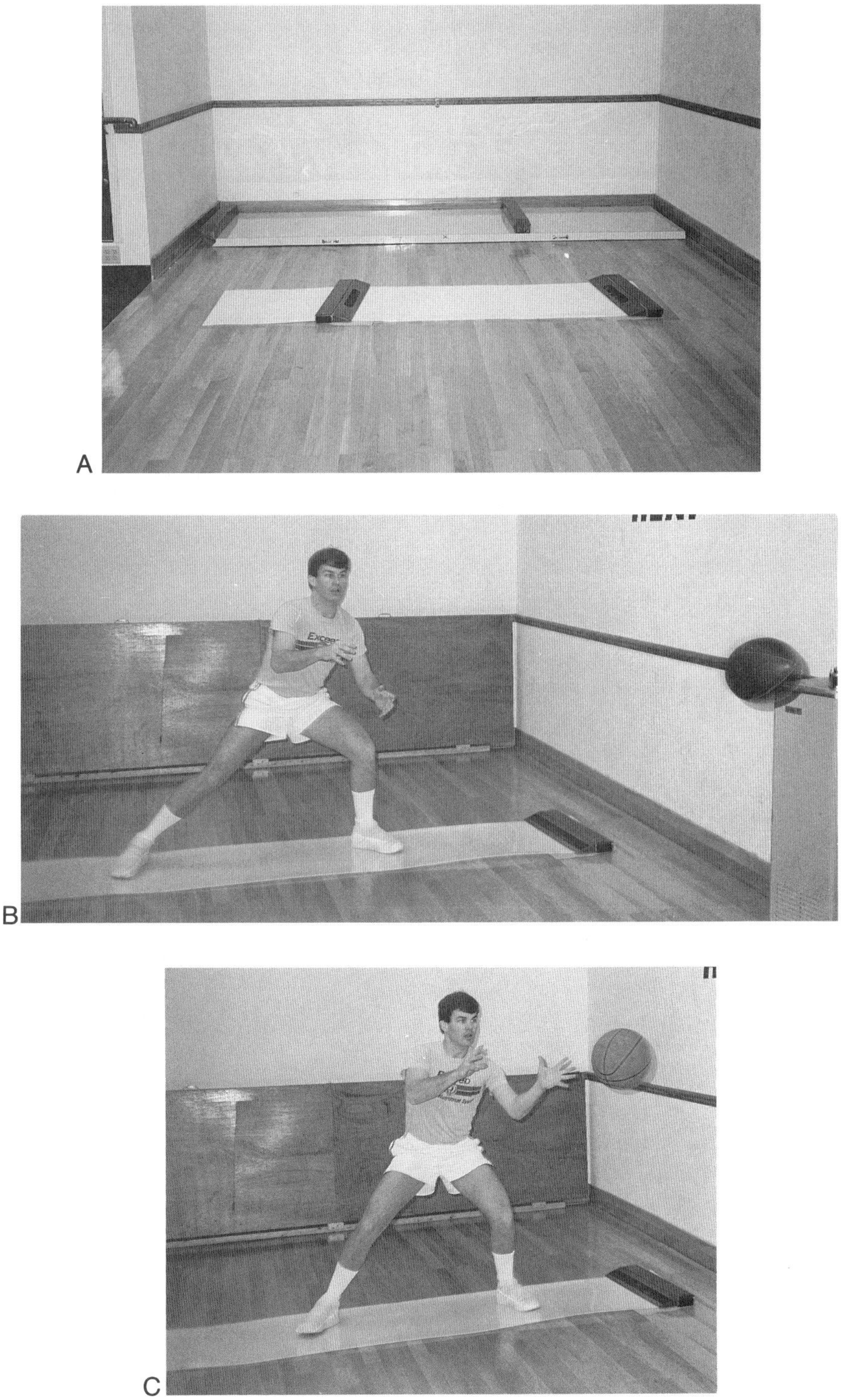

Fig. 4-7. Slide board/Euroglide sport-specific rehabilitation. **(A)** The slide board and Euroglide can be used as rehabilitation devices or as conditioning tools. Sport-specific rehabilitation may also be performed using the athlete's respective sports implements, as demonstrated with **(B)** a football and **(C)** a basketball.

productive, as increased time is spent in the amortization phase and energy is lost as heat. Other Soviet researchers[43,44] reported optimal results from a height of 320 centimeters (10 feet); however, they also reported that motivation was a problem and considerable coaxing was required to get the athlete to jump. While height is one consideration, the quality of the jump is most important. The response should be powerful with full body extension at push off regardless of the box height (Table 4-12). Therefore, most learning should take place at heights no greater than 24 inches, while advanced training should not exceed 42 inches.

Because depth jumping produces high stress reactions on the tendons and muscles, certain precautions must be followed to prevent injuries from occurring:

A

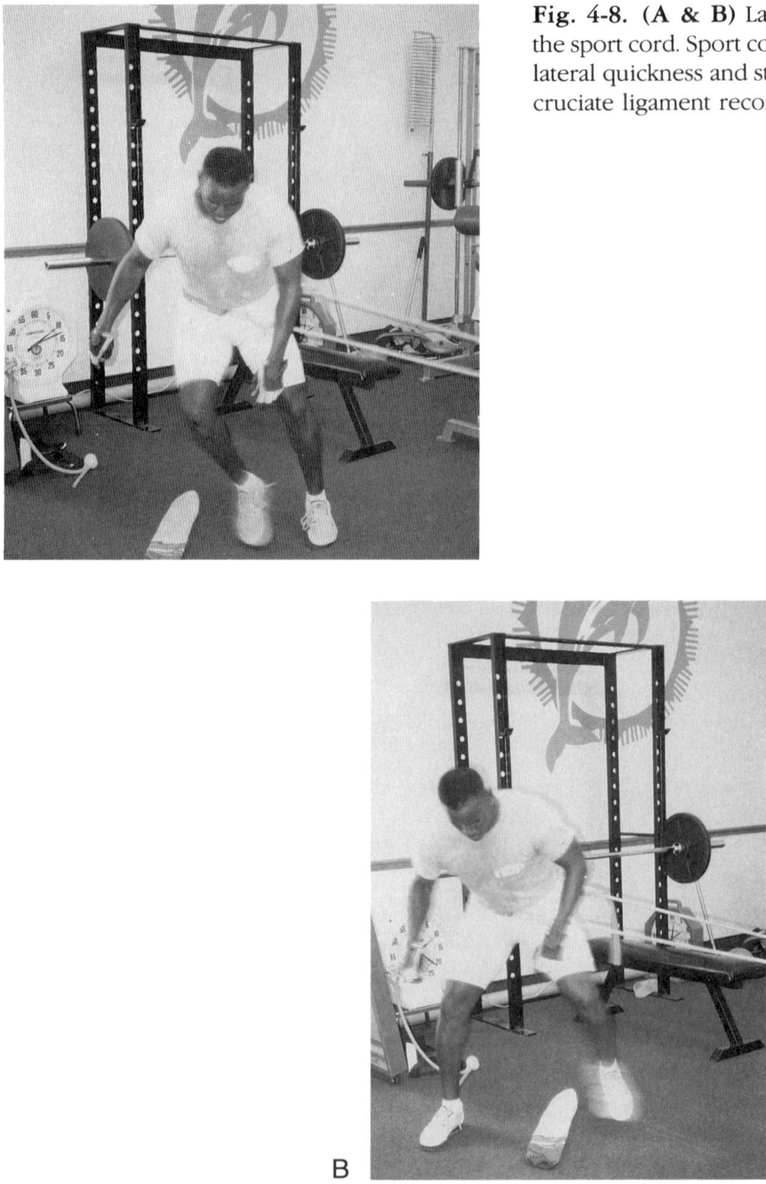

B

Fig. 4-8. (A & B) Lateral movement exercises utilizing the sport cord. Sport cord exercises are used for increasing lateral quickness and stability in the postoperative anterior cruciate ligament reconstruction patient.

1. Before depth jump training is initiated, low to moderate in-place jump training should be performed.
2. Initial depth jump height should not exceed 24 inches.
3. Maximal depth jump height should not exceed 42 inches. (While some Soviet researchers used maximal box heights of 2.8 to 3.2 meters and obtained good improvement, the stress of such jumping can lead to both immediate and overuse type injuries.)
4. Depth jump training with weighted vests, belts, or dumbbell weights can be extremely stressful and therefore should be performed with great caution.

A

B

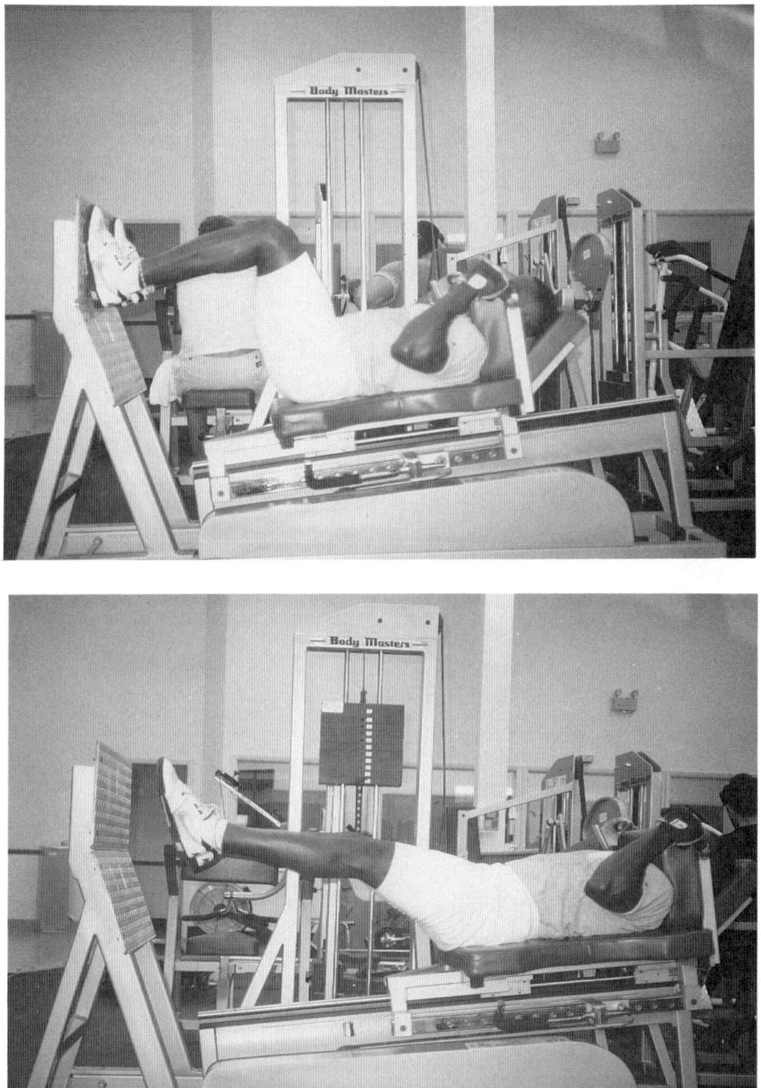

Fig. 4-9. (A & B) Leg press jumps. Such jumps offer the clinician a modified plyometric activity within a controlled environment.

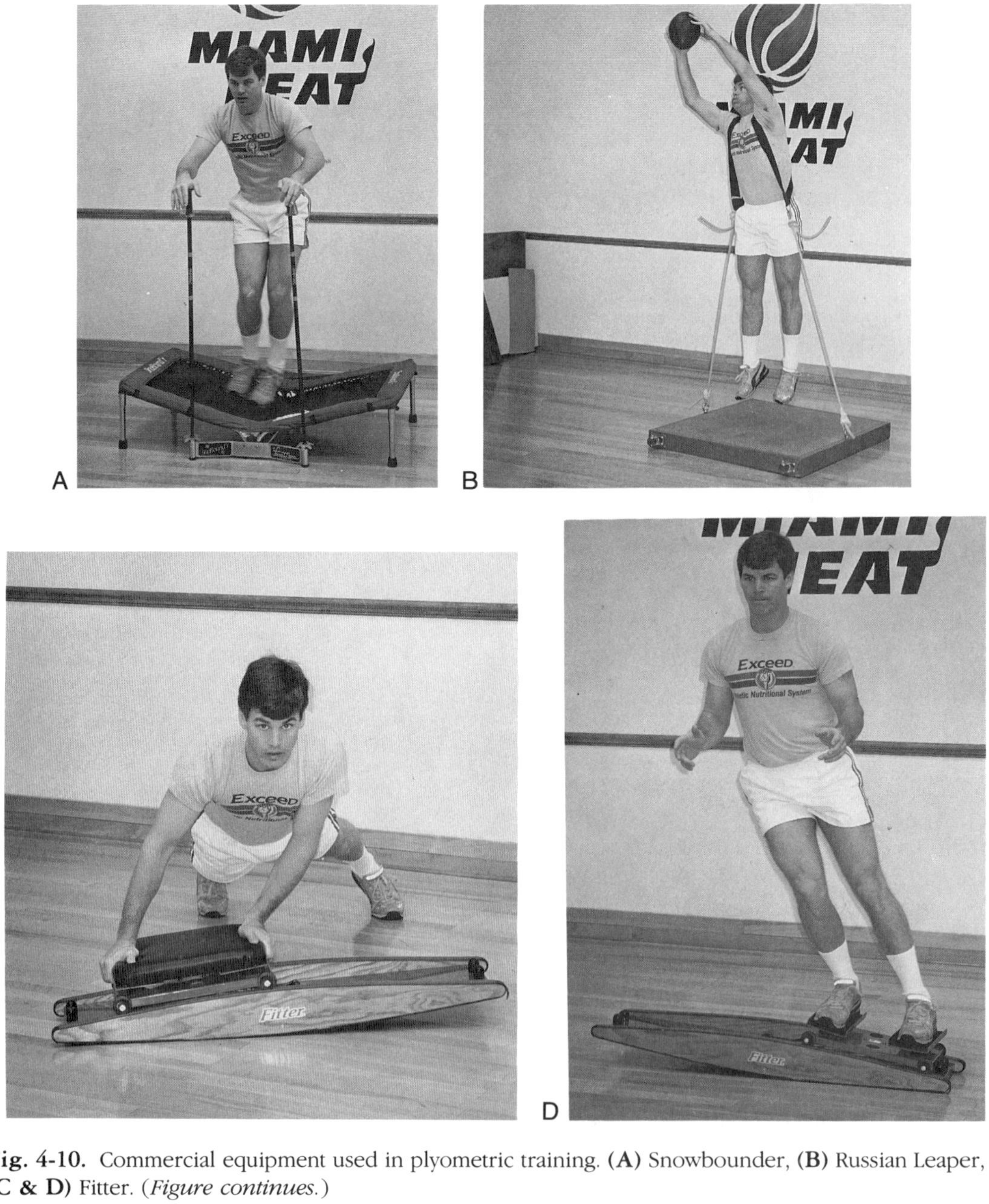

Fig. 4-10. Commercial equipment used in plyometric training. **(A)** Snowbounder, **(B)** Russian Leaper, **(C & D)** Fitter. (*Figure continues.*)

Figures 4-7 to 4-10 demonstrate other forms of plyometric type exercises for the lower quarter.

UPPER QUARTER TRAINING

While plyometric training is most often used to refer to jump training in the lower quarter, plyometric training can be applied to the upper quarter as well (Table 4-13, Fig. 4-11). Any exercise utilizing an eccentric prestretch followed by an explosive concentric contraction is plyometric in nature. Since the musculature of the upper quarter possesses the same physiologic characteristics as the lower extremity, various forms of exercise can be used to exploit the stretch reflex. A simple exercise program consisting of pushups can be used

E

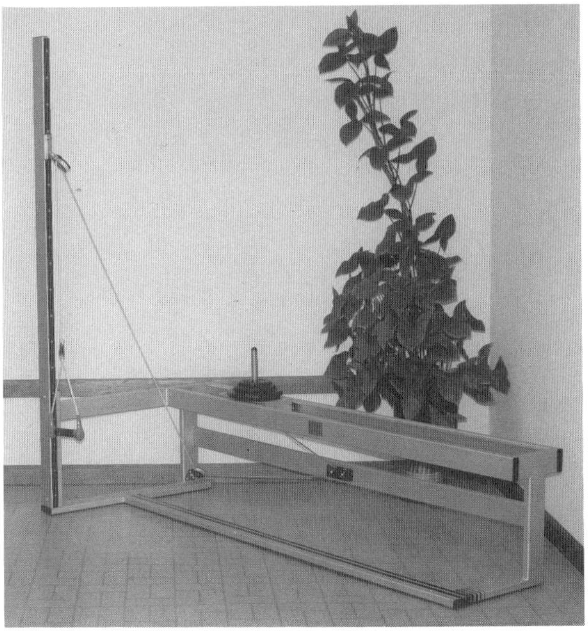

Fig. 4-10 (*Continued*). **(E)** Impulse inertial exerciser.

Table 4-13. Upper Quarter Plyometrics

Medicine ball
Chest pass standing
Chest pass kneeling
One hand
Two hand
Soccer throw
Tubing
IR/ER plyometrics
Diagonal movement patterns
Pushup program
On box
Two hand drops—rebounds
Two hand "clappers"
Alternate hand side to side
One hand pushup
Impulse Inertial Exerciser

to develop power in the shoulder girdle region. The medicine ball is a valuable tool in the upper quarter plyometric program.[45,46] Surgical tubing and the Impulse Inertial Exercise System can also be used to reproduce the stretch-shortening response.

TRUNK PROGRESSION

The trunk plays an equally important role in athletic movement. In addition to controlling posture, the trunk serves as the vital link for the transferrence of forces from the lower extremity to the upper extremity. This force transfer is a common occurrence and necessary in the throwing and racquet sports. Some of the equipment utilized with trunk plyometrics include the medicine ball,

Table 4-14. Trunk Progression

Leg throw downs
Straight
Diagonal
Cable pulleys
High pulley/low pulley
Alternating
Stretching stick
Right/left rotations
Right/left sidebends
Diagonals

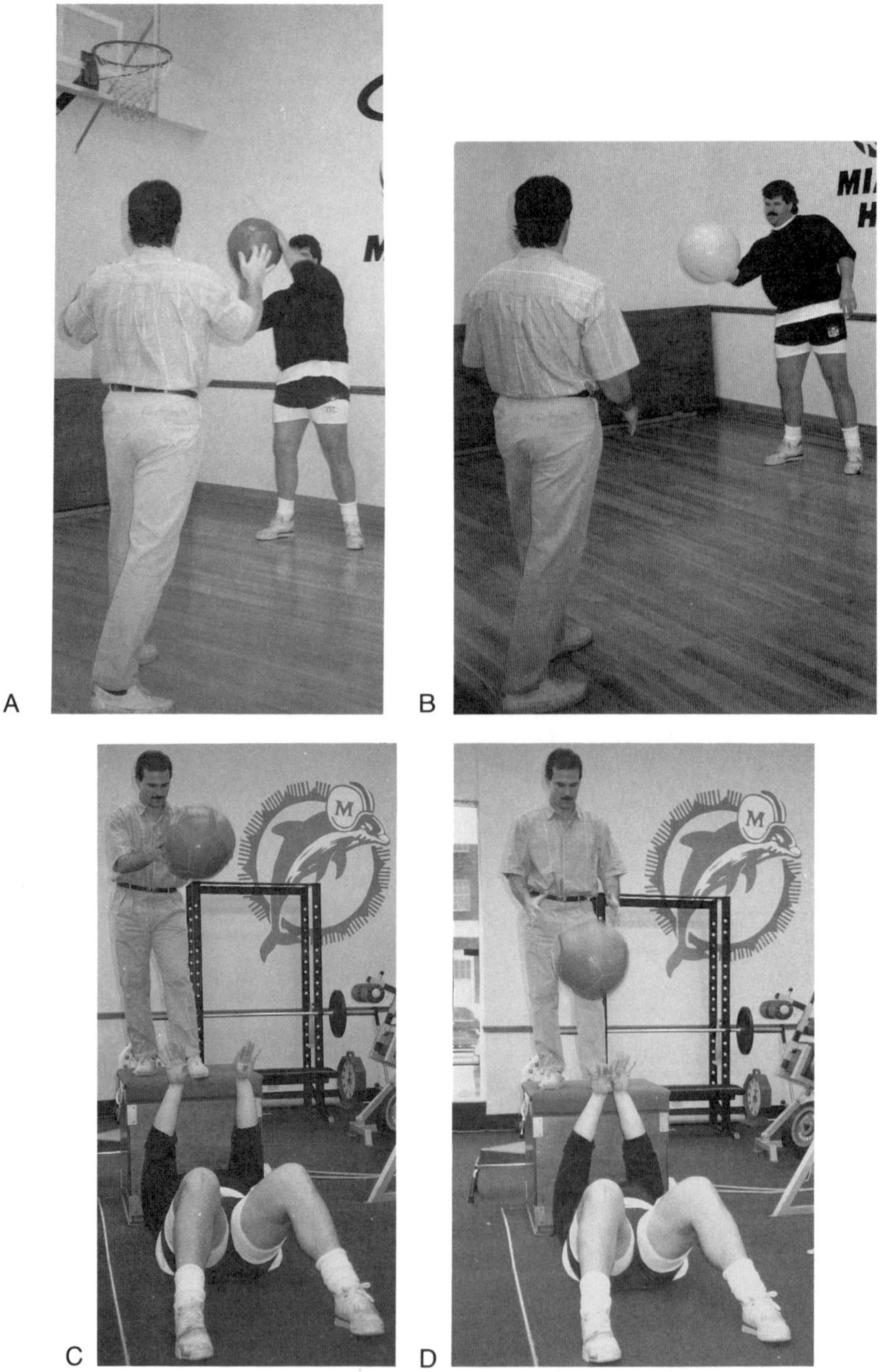

Fig. 4-11. Upper body medicine ball exercises may begin with **(A)** two hand throws, progress to **(B)** one hand throws, and eventually to sport-specific activities. **(C & D)** Pass blocking drills for football offensive linemen.

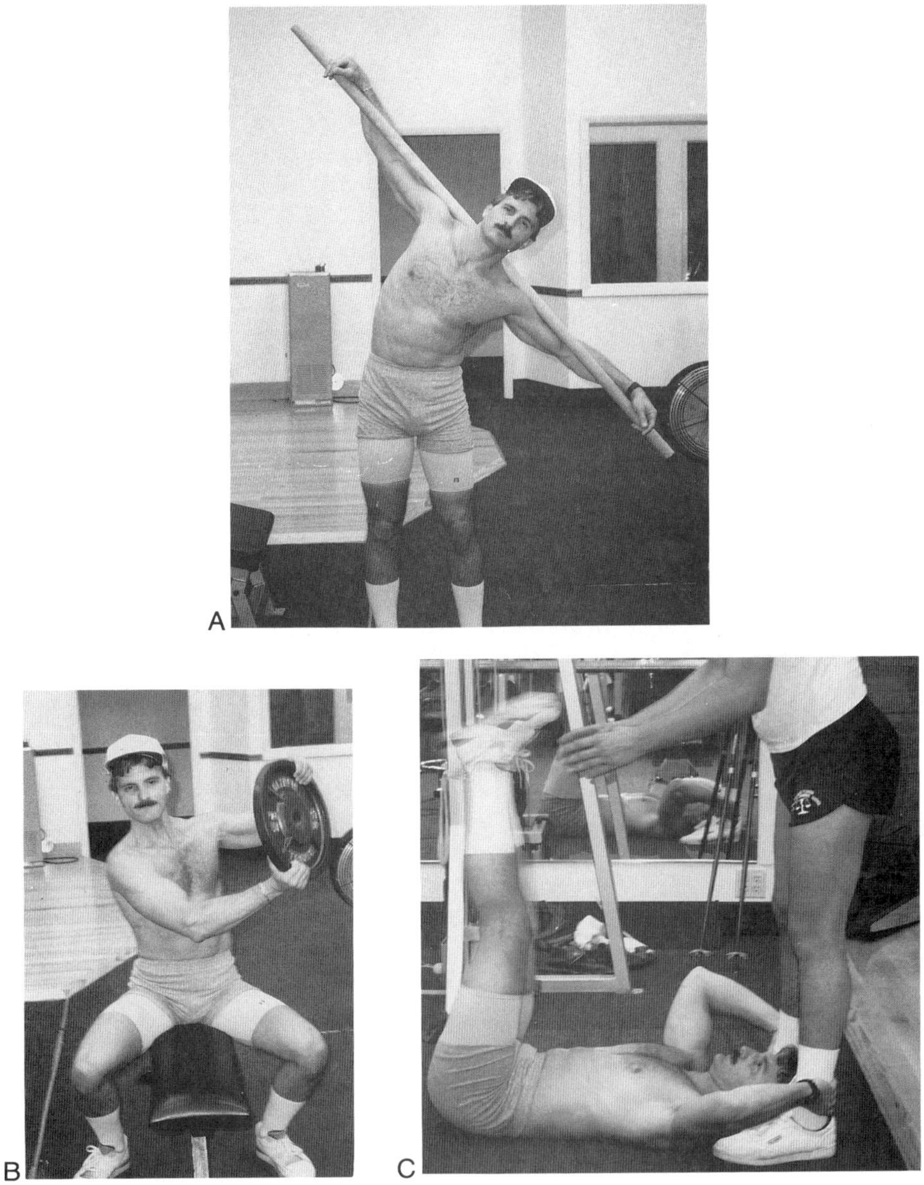

Fig. 4-12. Additional equipment used for trunk plyometrics include **(A)** the stretching stick, **(B)** weight plates, and even manual resistance, as demonstrated by **(C)** throw downs.

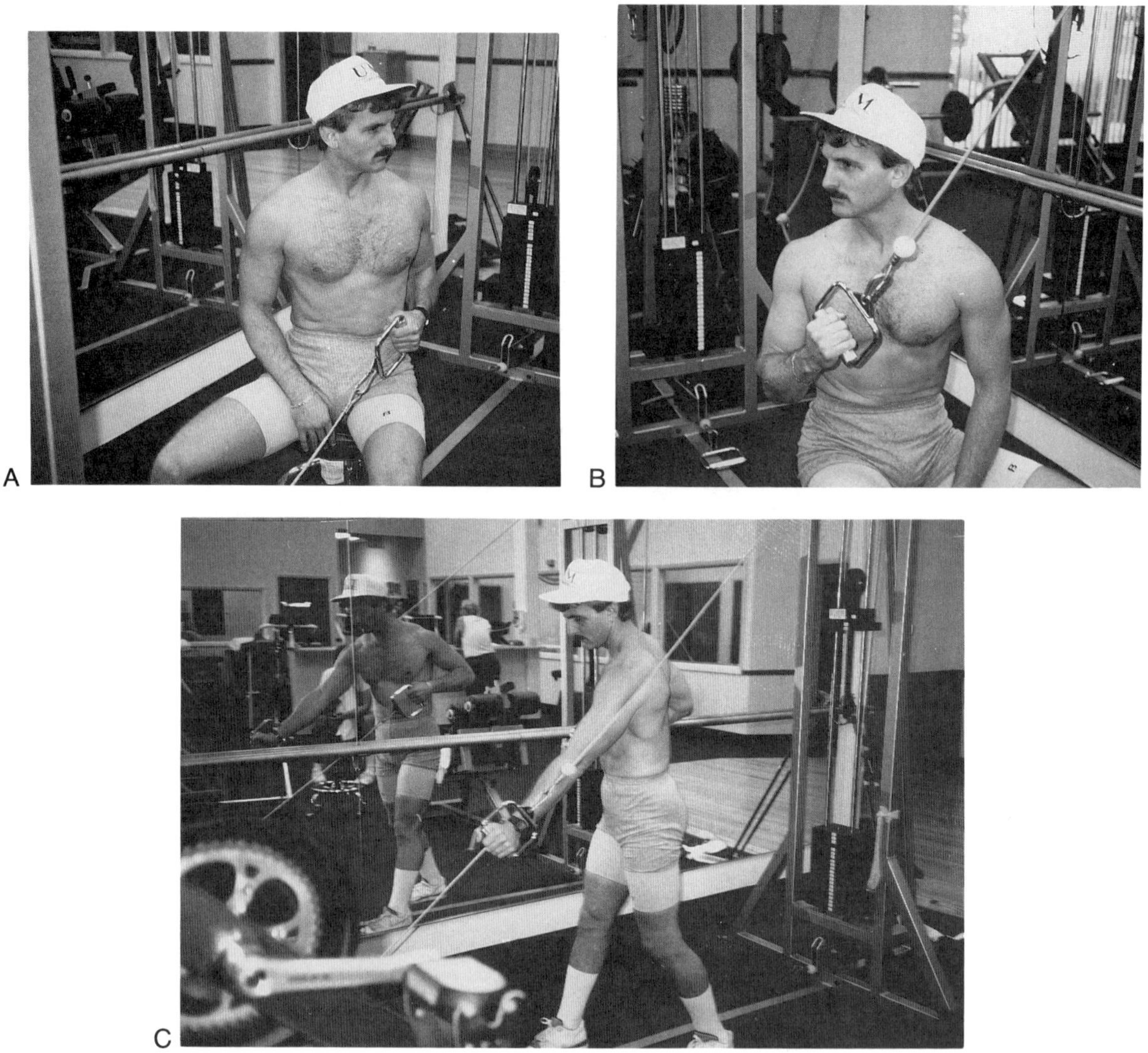

Fig. 4-13. Trunk exercises with cables. Cable exercises can be performed using **(A)** a low pulley, **(B)** high pulley, or **(C)** alternating pulleys.

weight plates, stretching stick, and a cable pulley system (Table 4-12, Figs. 4-12 to 4-15).

PLYOMETRICS AND INJURY REHABILITATION

It has been demonstrated that if injury rehabilitation is inadequate, the risk for reinjury is increased.[47] Before an athlete is given clearance for return to a particular sport, the body must be able to withstand the forces that the sport will demand.[27] Therefore, it is essential that the rehabilitation program include both concentric and eccentric components as soon as possible.[48,49] The principle of training specificity and sport specificity must also receive consideration during the design and development of the rehabilitation program.[50] Finally, the skeletal and neuromuscular systems must be functionally trained to prepare

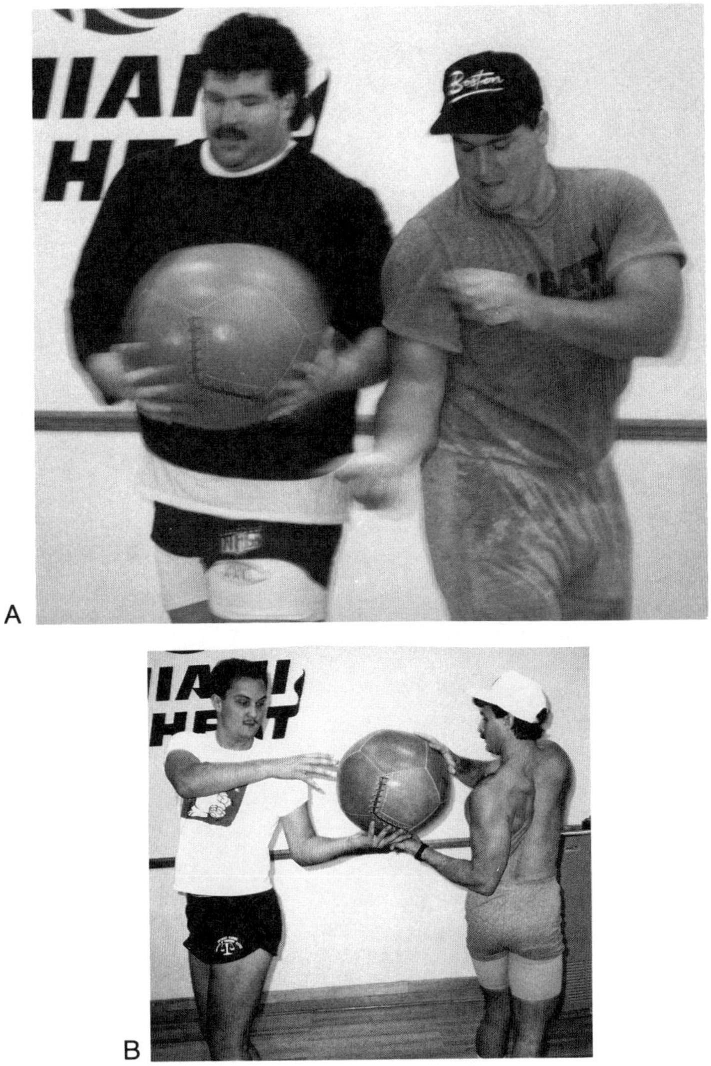

Fig 4-14. Medicine ball partner exercises demonstrate **(A)** rotations and **(B)** figure 8s.

the athlete for the specific demands required for returning to that respective sport.[51] The injury rehabilitation process serves to progressively remodel and re-educate the injured tissues in the shortest, safest period of time.

In early rehabilitation, above all else, the primary concern is the time constraints of soft tissue healing.[51] Stanitski[33] states, "Healing is a function not of technology, but rather of biology." Although we do not have control over this factor, we do have control over modeling and remodeling of the injured tissues. Once the time constraints of soft tissue healing are no longer a concern, the next step is to analyze the specific movement pattern so that it may be broken down into component parts.

There are many factors that may contribute to overuse tendon injuries.[52] One classification system groups the factors into either intrinsic or extrinsic. Intrinsic factors include malalignment, limb length discrepancy, muscular imbalance, and muscular insufficiency. Extrinsic factors include

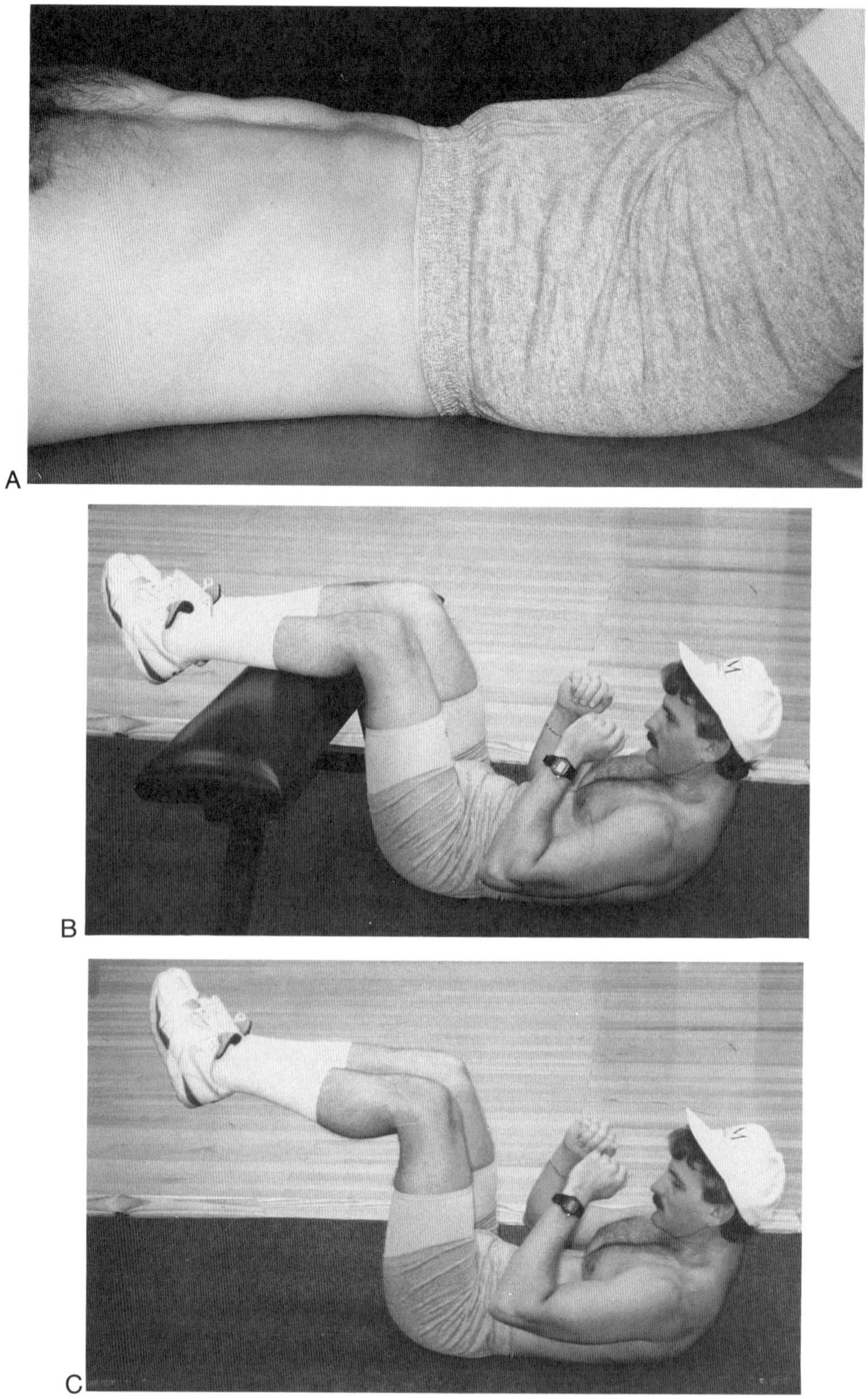

Fig. 4-15. The situp progression is illustrated in the following sequence: **(A)** pelvic tilts; **(B)** crunches with legs supported; **(C)** crunches with legs unsupported. (*Figure continues.*)

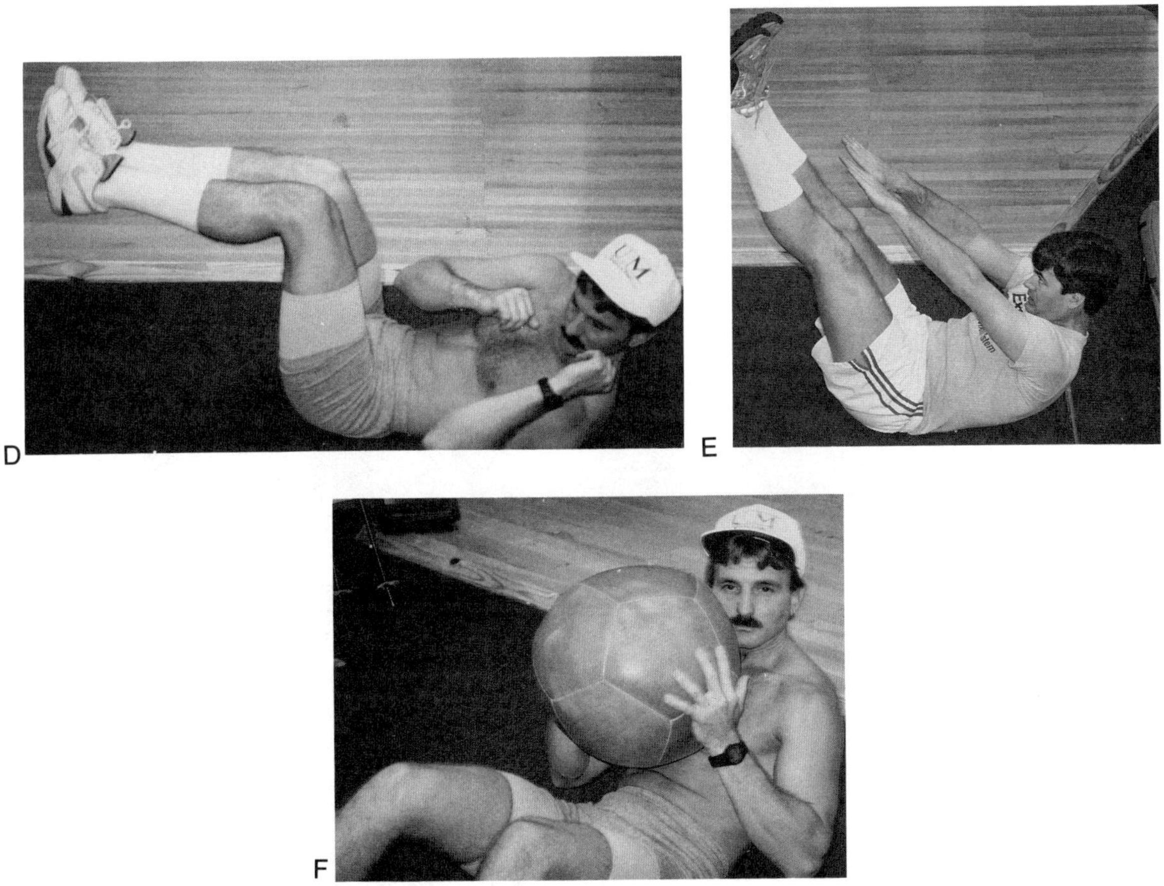

Fig. 4-15 (*Continued*). **(D)** Crunches with twist; **(E)** pike situps; **(F)** chest pass medicine ball situps. (*Figure continues.*)

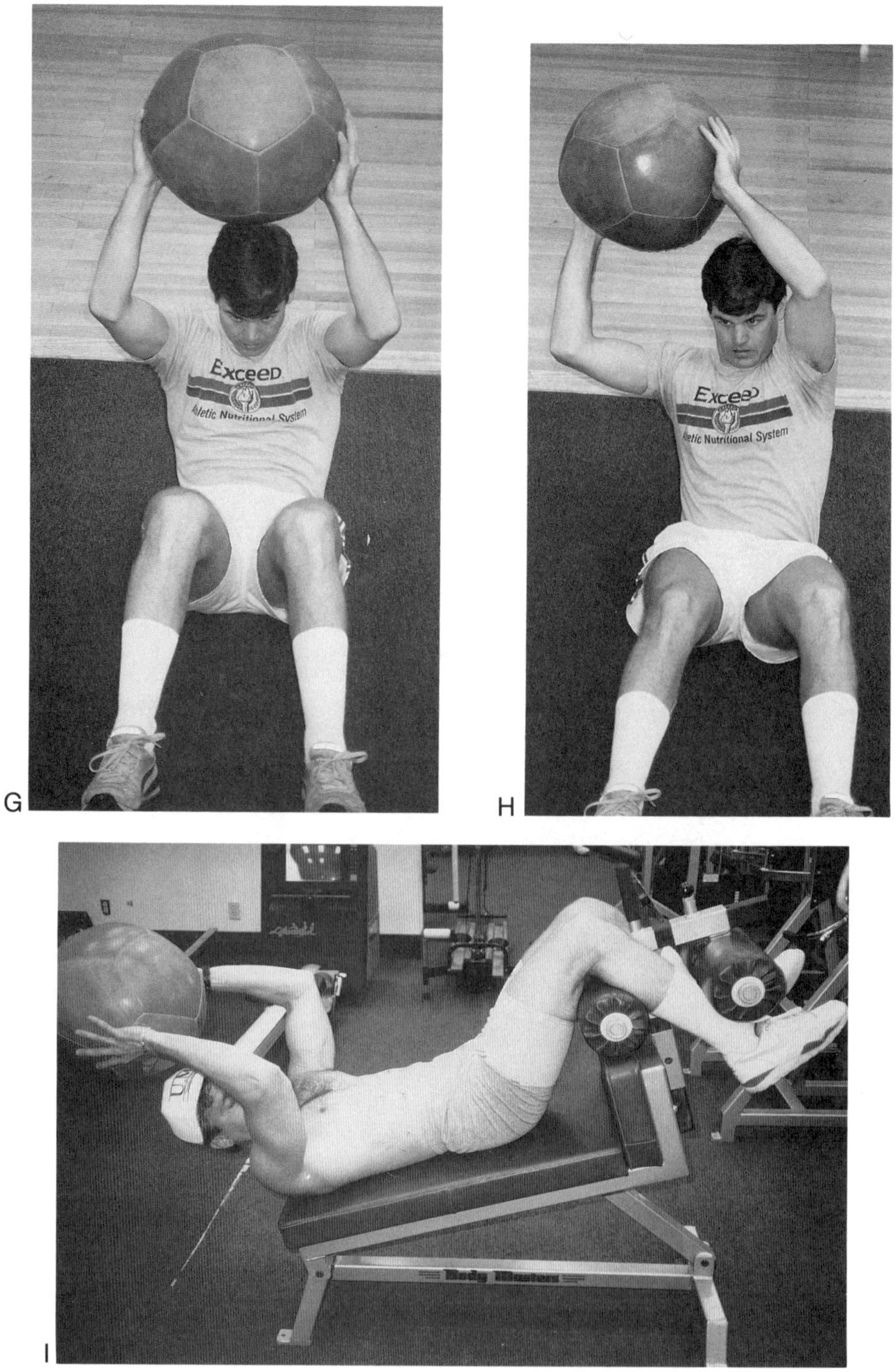

Fig. 4-15 (*Continued*). **(G)** Overhead pass medicine ball situps; **(H)** right/left overhead pass medicine ball situps; and **(I)** incline medicine ball pass situps.

surface area, footwear and equipment, environmental conditions, and training error.[48] Intrinsic factors can be detected during the preparticipation clearance evaluation while extrinsic factors are inexcusable. Extrinsic factors are all factors of consideration when the rehabilitation program is being designed.

Before return to competitive play is allowed, the athlete must successfully demonstrate each component of skill. In the early part of the rehabilitation program, plyometrics can be implemented, but with modifications and special equipment. Some of the special equipment utilized is the CMC Shuttle 2000, impulse inertial exerciser, water jets, SPORT cord tubing, bath towels, fitter, and isotonic weight equipment. The CMC Shuttle 2000 provides the rehabilitation specialist with a transitional piece of equipment. The shuttle's versatility is an attractive feature, while its horizontal loading mechanism allows the shuttle to be used throughout the rehabilitation process. The inertial exerciser allows for a progressive weight and speed overload for concentric-eccentric loading. Water jet utilization eliminates the effects of gravity, but incorporates open chain rapid stretching. SPORT cord exercises are limited only by the creativeness of the therapist. Rapid fire explosive muscle contractions can be performed against the resistance of the cords. SPORT cords can also be used in swimming to improve power during push off in the flip turn. Towels afford the therapist a good alternative for controlling the magnitude and direction of the rapid stretch. Remember, the speed of the stimulus is more important than the magnitude. The Euroglide or slide board can be utilized in sport-specific training. While sliding, the athlete can focus on swinging a racquet or catching a ball. This takes the conscious mind out of the act and does not allow the athlete to think about the sliding activity. In turn this will prevent secondary gaurding of the injured region and allow a progressive increase in stress to the injured region. Progression is controlled by increasing the distance covered during the slide, or increasing the number of repetitions within a certain time period. A horizontal leg press can also be used when initiating early plyometrics.

Early phase plyometrics can be done in a well controlled environment as long as it does not contradict the constraints of soft tissue healing. In fact, it is essential for the successful return of the athletes to their respective athletic environments.

CONCLUSION

Currently, plyometric training has both advocates and opponents. Empirical testimony on behalf of plyometric training suggests improved performance, while its opposition contends that plyometric training increases the risk of injury. It should be emphasized that plyometrics can be dangerous if placed in the hands of inexperienced supervision. Theoretically, a successful plyometric program should be sequentially designed, follow an established strength base, and be supervised by a person with a thorough scientific and practical understanding of both functional biomechanics and functional training progressions.

We believe that a successful plyometric program can be realized without placing the athlete in an environment that invites an increased risk for training injuries. This is possible, but only if common sense is exercised and the necessary individual modifications are made and adhered to. Before complete acceptance of plyometric training can be expected the following are necessary:

1. Universal testing and data collection procedures must be established so that safe but effective normative data can be developed.
2. Future well controlled studies must be conducted which address the benefit-injury risk factor ratio.
3. Everyone wishing to incorporate this form of training must make it their responsibility to understand the scientific and practical principles involved. This is necessary to ensure that plyometric training does not predispose athletes to either traumatic or overuse injuries.
4. Documented objective pre- to post-test comparative scores must be translated into improved skill and sports performance.

We empirically conclude that scientifically designed plyometric programs, geared towards the needs and specific limitations of each individual, can serve to provide the sports performance specialist with a viable, practical training form for developing additional measurable power.

A plyometric training program can include a large variety of different exercises with the only limitation being the creativeness of the program organizer. Since year round training can lead to boredom and lack of motivation, every effort should be made to provide variety in the training/rehabilitation program. Program variety can be manipulated with different pieces of equipment or kinds of movement performed. Continued motivation and an organized progression are the keys to success. Failing to plan is planning to fail.

REFERENCES

1. Chu D, Plummer L: The language of plyometrics. NSCA Journal 6:30, 1984
2. Wilt F: Plyometrics-what it is and how it works. Athletic Journal 55b:76, 1975
3. Verhoshanski Y, Chornonson G: Jump exercises in sprint training. Track and Field Quarterly 9:1909, 1967
4. Vermil A: Game day inseason training in the Chicago Bulls. NSCA Journal 11:47, 1989
5. Asmussen E, Bonde-Peterson F: Storage of elastic energy in skeletal muscles in man. Acta Physiol Scand 91:385, 1974
6. Bosco C, Komi PV: Potentiation of the mechanical behavior of the human skeletal muscle through prestretching. Acta Physiol Scand 106:467, 1979
7. Cavagna G, Saibene F, Margaria R: Effect of negative work on the amount of positive work performed by an isolated muscle. J Appl Physiol 20:157, 1965
8. Enoka RM: Neuromechanical Basis of Kinesiology. Human Kinetics, Champaign, 1988
9. Lundin P: A review of plyometric training. NSCA Journal 7:69, 1985
10. Rowinski M: The role of eccentric exercise. Biodex Corporation, Pro Clinica Inc., pp. 1–8, 1988
11. Cavagna GA, Dusman B, Margaria R: Positive work done by a previously stretched muscle. J Appl Physiol 24:21, 1968
12. Komi P, Buskirk E: Effects of eccentric and concentric muscle conditioning on tension and electrical activity of human muscle. Ergonomics 15:417, 1972
13. Thomas DW: Plyometrics—more than the stretch reflex. NSCA Journal 10:49, 1988
14. Komi PV, Bosco C: Utilization of stored elastic energy in leg extensor muscles by men and women. Med Sci Sports Exerc 10:261, 1978
15. Komi PV: Physiological and biomechanical correlates of muscle function: Effects of muscle structure and stretch-shortening cycle on force and speed. p. 81. In Terjung RL (ed): Exercise and Sport Sciences Reviews. Collamore Press, Lexington, 1984
16. Stauber WT: Eccentric action of muscles: Physiology, injury, and adaptation. p. 157. In Pandolf KB (ed): Exercise and Sport Sciences Reviews. Williams & Wilkins, Baltimore, 1989
17. Chu D: Conditioning/plyometrics. Paper presented at 10th Annual Sports Medicine Team Concept Conference, San Francisco, CA, December 1989
18. Enoka RM: Muscle strength and its development. New perspectives. Sports Med 6:146, 1988
19. Hakkwan K, Komi PV: Electromyographic changes during strength training and detraining. Med Sci Sports Exerc 15:455, 1983
20. Michielli DW: Skeletal muscle and its adaptation to exercise training. p. 1. In Nudel DB(ed): Pediatric Sports Medicine. PMA, New York, 1989
21. Sale DG: Neural adaption to resistance training. Med Sci Sports Exerc suppl. 5: S135, 1988
22. Zajac FE, Gordon ME: Determining muscle's force and action in multi-articular movements. p. 187. In Pandolf KB (ed): Exercise and Sport Sciences Reviews. Vol. 17. Williams & Wilkins, Baltimore, 1989
23. Hortobagyi T (ed): Theoretical and Methodological Basis of Training Planning with Special Considerations within a Microcycle. National Strength and Conditioning Association, Lincoln, 1989
24. Matveyev L: Fundamentals of Sports Training. Progress Publishers, Moscow, 1977
25. Bielik E, Chu DA, Costello F et al: Roundtable. Practical considerations for utilizing plyometrics. Part I: NSCA Jounral 8:14, 1985, and Part II: NSCA Journal 8:14, 1986
26. Rasch PJ, Grabiner MD, Gregor RJ, Garhammer J: Kinesiology and Applied Anatomy. 7th Ed. Lea & Febiger, Philadelphia, 1989
27. Wallis EL, Logan GA: Figure Improvement and Body Conditioning Through Exercise. Prentice Hall, Englewood Cliffs, 1964
28. Javorek I: Plyometrics. NSCA Journal 11:52, 1989
29. Chu D: Plyometric Exercise, NSCA Journal 6:56, 1984
30. Jensen C: Pertinent facts about warming. Athletic Journal 56:72, 1975

31. Radcliffe JC, Farentinos RC: Plyometrics Explosive Power Training. 2nd Ed. Human Kinetics, Champaign, 1985
32. Rook DS, Micheli LJ: Musculoskeletal Assessment and Training: The Young Athlete. P. 641. In Micheli LJ (ed): Clinics in Sports Medicine. WB Saunders, Philadelphia, 1988
33. Stanitski CL: Common injuries in preadolescents and adolescent athletes. Recommendations for prevention. Sports Med 7:32, 1989
34. Zauner CW, Maksud MG, Melichna J: Physiological considerations in training young athletes. Sports Med 8:15, 1989
35. Brody TA: Weight training related injuries. Am J Sports Med 10:1, 1982
36. Fleck SJ, Kraemer WJ: Designing Resistance Training Programs, Human Kinetics, Champaign, 1987
37. Jacobson BH, Kulling FA: Effect of resistive weight training in pre-pubescents. J Orthop Sports Phys Ther 11:96, 1989
38. Bobbert MF: Drop jumping as a training method for jumping ability. Sports Med 9:7, 1990
39. Duda M: Plyometrics: A legitimate form of power training? Phys Sports Med 16:213, 1988
40. Birrer RB, Levine R: Performance parameters in children and adolescent athletes. Sports Med 4:211, 1987
41. O'Neill D, Micheli LJ: Overuse injuries in the young athlete. p. 591. In Micheli LF (ed): Clinics in Sports Medicine. WB Saunders, Philadelphia, 1988
42. Verhoshanski V: Are depth jumps useful? Track and Field 12:9, 1967
43. Dunsenev CI: Strength training of jumpers. Track and Field Quarterly Review 82:4, 1982
44. Dunsenev CI: Strength training for jumpers. Soviet Sports Review 14:2, 1979
45. Chu D: Plyometric Exercises with the Medicine Ball. Bittersweet Publishing Co, Livermore, 1989
46. Lorette L: Medicine Ball Exercise Cycles. Communication Press, Austin, 1983
47. Edgerton VR: Neuromuscular adaptation to power and endurance work. Can J Appl Sports Sci 1:49, 1976
48. Renstrom P, Johnson R: Overuse injuries in sports. A review. Sports Med 2:316, 1985
49. Stanish WD, Rubinovich RM, Curwin S: Eccentric exercise in chronic tendinitis. Clin Orthop Rel Res 208:65, 1986
50. Rutherford OM: Muscular coordination and strength training. Implications for injury rehabilitation. Sports Med 5:196, 1988
51. Mangine RE: Functional rehabilitation. Clinical concepts for rehabilitation. Paper presented at 1985 Cincinnati Sports Medicine Conference.
52. Curwin S, Stanish W: Tendinitis: Its Etiology and Treatment. Collamore Press, Lexington, 1984
53. Schmidt RA: Motor Control and Learning. 2nd Ed. Human Kinetics, Champaign, IL, 1988
54. Plyometric Training: Understanding and Coaching Power Development for Sport (videotape). National Strength and Conditioning Association, PO Box 81410, Lincoln, NE 68501
55. Chu D: Pliometrics: Dynamic Conditioning and Training (videotape). Championship Books, PO Box 1166, ISU Station, Ames, Iowa

5
Inertial Training Concepts

Inertial loading to the musculoskeletal system was initially introduced as a clinical device in the form of Impulse unit (Engineering Marketing Associates [EMA], Newnan, GA) (Fig. 5-1) in 1985. The Impulse was designed by the team of Tom McLaughlin, biomechanist, Ron Peyton, P.T., Bill McLeod, Ph.D., biomechanist, and Steve Davison, engineer. The Impulse system, also known as the Inertial Exercise System (IES), represents new technology that offers multiple potential applications in orthopaedic and neuromuscular rehabilitation as well as performance and prevention training. In the early 1970s, the introduction of isokinetics produced a situation whereby technologic advancement preceded both clinical understanding and research development. Today, a parallel situation exists with inertial exercise.

Statements by Davies (course notes, Atlanta, GA, 1988) and Biodex[1] assert that as high as 85 percent of human motion is either accelerational or decelerational. With this in mind, inertial loading causes the muscles to rapidly and repetitively behave in both accelerational and decelerational (eccentric) conditions. In addition, the Impulse system incorporates multiplanar, high speed movement patterns with functional eccentric responses. The concept of "functional" eccentrics is described by McLeod (course notes, Charleston, SC, 1986) as involving three elements: (1) large forces; (2) short duration; and (3) stretch reflex modulated.

The concept of specificity of exercise with respect to functional speeds of motion must be clarified. While the isokinetic terminology classifies high speed as more than 180 degrees per second, actual functional demands may easily exceed the top threshold of isokinetic dynamometers at 400 to 500 degrees per second and reach as high as 10,000 degrees per second[2,3] (and McLeod course notes). Such pronounced speed differences result from the addition of potential energy through eccentrics, muscular prestretch, and summation of multiple segmental momentum. Grillner[4] contends that the reflex loop and proprioceptive feedback are too slow to compensate for most high load demands encountered in functional activities. Grillner postulates that the primary mechanism for necessary force adjustments result from the natural viscoelasticity of the muscle and connective tissue.

Joint forces are the result of muscular, gravitational, and inertial components and are subject to the summation of momentum through kinetic chain principles. The form of resistance involved in the Impulse unit simulates the momentum changes that occur functionally, by use of a weight plate mounted on a horizontally sliding track (Fig. 5-2). The effects of gravity on the weight are virtually eliminated due to its linear motion and mechanical support from the machine's frame; meanwhile, minimal frictional resistance is encountered. The weight is accelerated into motion with concentric activity; inertia is overcome (see the section *Biophysical Principles and Applications*) and is "caught" by eccentric activity of the same muscle or group of muscles. The *catch* phase is interposed in a cyclic pattern between one concentric contraction and the next successive one— a pattern that closely resembles the biophysical events of the stretch-shorten cycle.[5] The cyclic pat-

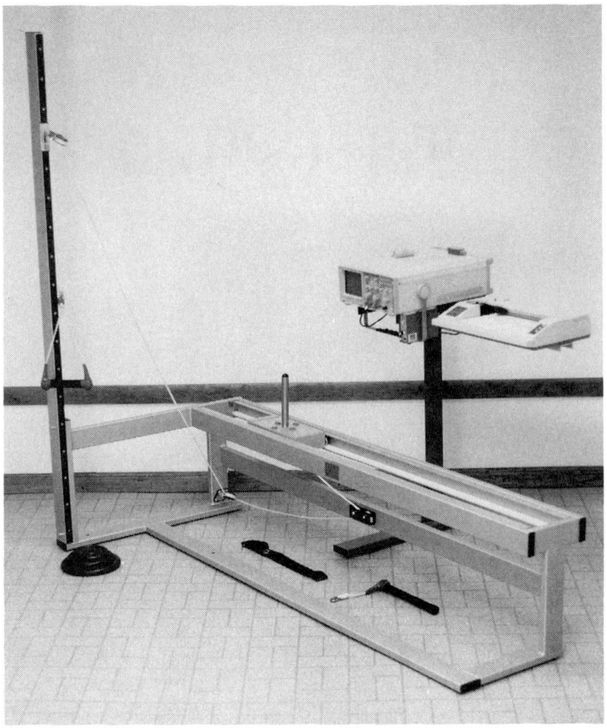

Fig. 5-1. Impulse system.

tern produced by the inertial loading incorporates selective loading of the series elastic component (SEC) with potential energy. By definition, a repetition on the Impulse system is the period from one eccentric catch to the next successive eccentric response. While inertial exercise repetitions are admittedly difficult to describe and to conceive without the physical experience, a starting point for understanding the complex series of movements must be offered. Motion first occurs from a discrete position in a select plane of movement, called initial position (IP), and an arc of motion is completed to the final position (FP). As the subject's control improves through neuromuscular adjustments, the IP and FP become fixed points as does the arc of motion (Fig. 5-3).

One feature of inertial loading that is unique when compared with other common forms of muscle loads (i.e., isotonics, isokinetics) is the existence of a relatively brief, but quieter muscular phase that can be called the *coast* phase. During this phase, interposed between one concentric and the succeeding eccentric response, the weight slides at a fixed speed across the track. Applying the definition of isokinetics as fixed speed, variable resistance training, the coast phase resembles isokinetic-like conditions. The possibility that inertial loading may require not only concentric and eccentric muscle activity but also isokinetic loading is a clinically exciting concept that formed the research hypothesis for a pilot study performed in 1987 (see the section *Proposed Inertial Loading*). Certainly, further research on this specific area of inertial exercise is warranted.

As discussed by Bosco and Komi,[6] the degree of elastic energy buildup is directly related to the velocity of the preceding stretching force. Inertial loading is capable of producing rapid stretching effects within each movement cycle, or repetition. Inertial loading, with its combined short duration eccentric responses and functional speeds, will depend on subconscious motor control mecha-

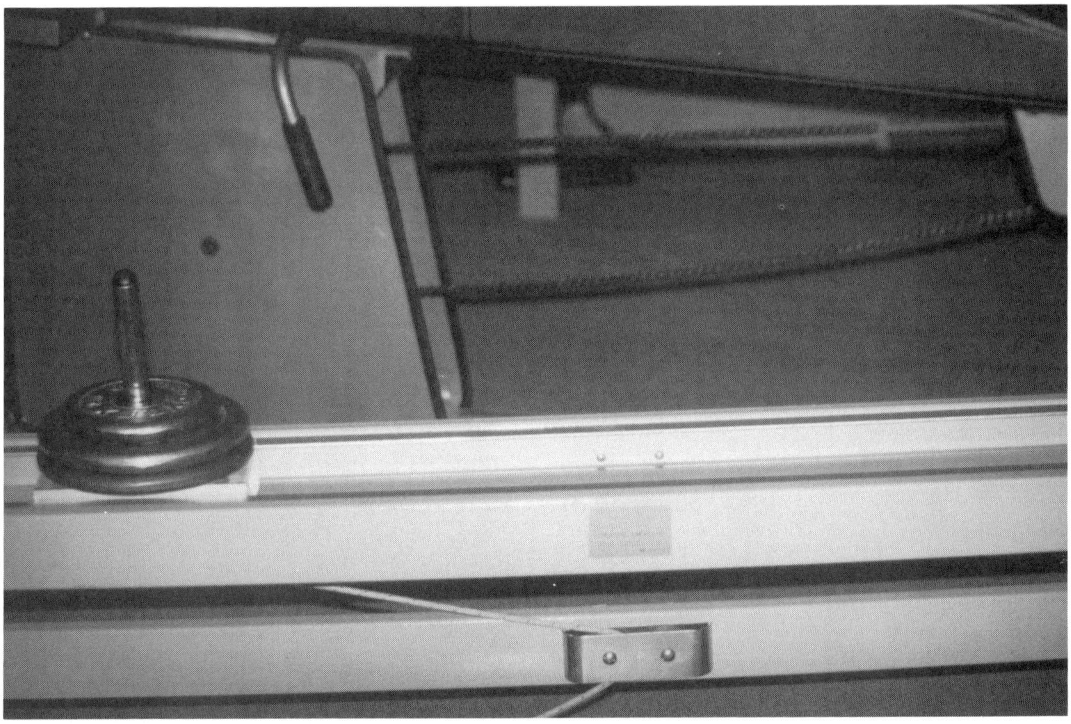

Fig. 5-2. Close-up of horizontally sliding platform.

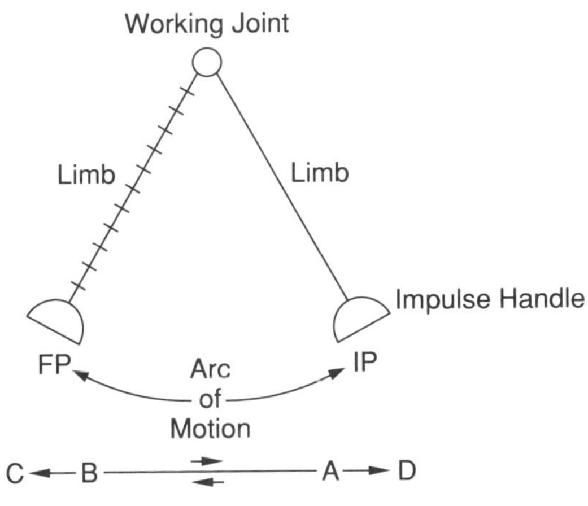

Fig. 5-3. Impulse repetition schematic. Repetition sequence: segment AB = concentric agonist; BC = eccentric agonist; concentric antagonist; BA = concentric antagonist, eccentric agonist; AD = eccentric agonist. Segments BC and AD represent the "catch" phase.

nisms. Hence, the Impulse may be considered a neuromuscular training device as opposed to being strictly a resistive exercise apparatus.

Due to the brief clinical history of inertial loading, the scientific literature contains few references regarding clinical usage, efficacy, or scientific bases. Chapman et al.[7] and Bober et al.[8] report effects of inertial type loads on the human muscular system. Chapman et al.[7] report that inertial loads are commonly required in many sports skills and daily activities. However, both Bober et al. and Chapman et al. implicate the importance of high speed eccentric stretch on facilitating concentric forces. Pertuzon and Bouisset[9] discussed muscular forces against inertial loads as being modified by joint influences into circular or rotational directions. Hakkinen and Komi[10] and Costill et al.[11] support the importance of mixed modes of exercise for optimal rehabilitation results, which the Impulse achieves through combined concentric and eccentric muscular activity at functional speeds.

BIOPHYSICAL PRINCIPLES AND APPLICATIONS

While clinicians may have infrequent opportunities to directly apply biophysical principles to clinical exercise situations, the IES affords numerous applications of straightforward biophysical and biomechanical formulas and relationships. The term *impulse* is a biophysical principle, defined as a unit of force applied over time (see schematic representation in Fig. 5-4). *Inertia*, meanwhile, is defined as the resistance of an object to a change in motion. Moment of inertia, is described as a resistance of an object to a change in angular motion. Simply stated, any change of motion, whether stopping or starting, or change in velocity is caused by a specific force. This relationship forms the basis for Isaac Newton's (1642–1727) three laws of motion.[12]

1. *Law of inertia*: Every body continues in its state of rest or uniform motion in a straight line except when it is compelled by external forces to change its state.
2. *Law of acceleration*: The rate of change of momentum of a body is proportional to the applied force, and takes place in the direction in which the force acts.
3. *Law of action-reaction*: To every action there is an equal and opposite reaction.

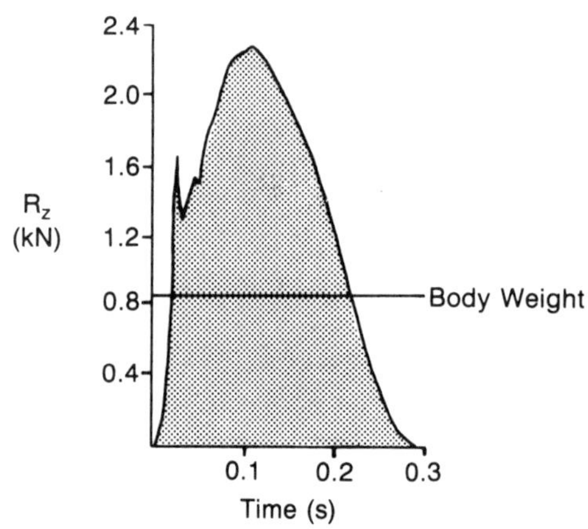

Fig. 5-4. Impulse curve (biophysical force of ground reaction). (From Enoka,[12] with permission.)

The law of acceleration refers to the concept of momentum, which is defined as the product of mass times velocity. Momentum is the form of resistance loading produced by the Impulse inertial unit, which serves to explain the multiple clinical differences that are encountered with inertial loading (see the section *Clinical Concepts*).

The definition of force is the product of mass times acceleration (A), where acceleration is characterized by the rate of change of velocity in the formula:

$$A = \frac{V_2 - V_1}{T}$$

where V_1 = starting velocity, V_2 = final velocity, and T = time. The element of work also applies to inertial loading and is defined as "force times distance," while power is equal to work divided by time.

All of the above formulas are easily applied to the use of the Impulse in the clinic. The weight placed on the sliding platform track of the Impulse acts as the mass, with muscular forces producing inertial and momentum changes and acceleration/deceleration as the velocity and direction of motion of sliding track are altered. Hence, inertial exercise involves clinical variables of weight and frequency rate (number of repetitions per given time period). Resultant force of the exercise is changed by increasing the weight with a set rate of movement, or increasing the rate of movement with the same weight.

An important area of biophysical application to the Impulse lies in the use of electronic transducers called accelerometers, which are readily coupled to Impulse setups. Accelerometers can monitor human motion with measurement of acceleration (or deceleration), the unit of measurement being expressed in "Gs," or 32 square feet per second. Balogun et al.,[13] Smith,[14] and Troup and Chapman[15] have all recommended the use of accelerometry in clinical practice. In fact, Steinhauf and Pawlus[16] conclude that neuromuscular testing through the use of accelerometry may be more sensitive in detecting changes in motion than either Cybex (isokinetic dynamometer) or high speed cinematography. Pertuzon and Bouisset[9] and Bergmaier and Neukomm[17] se-

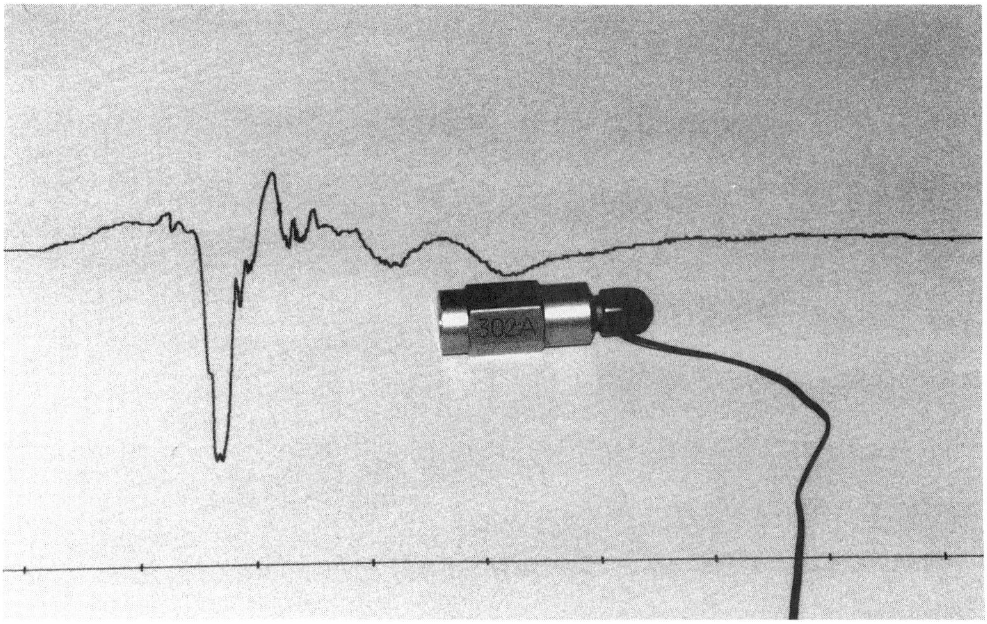

A

Fig. 5-5. (A & B) Accelerometry setup.

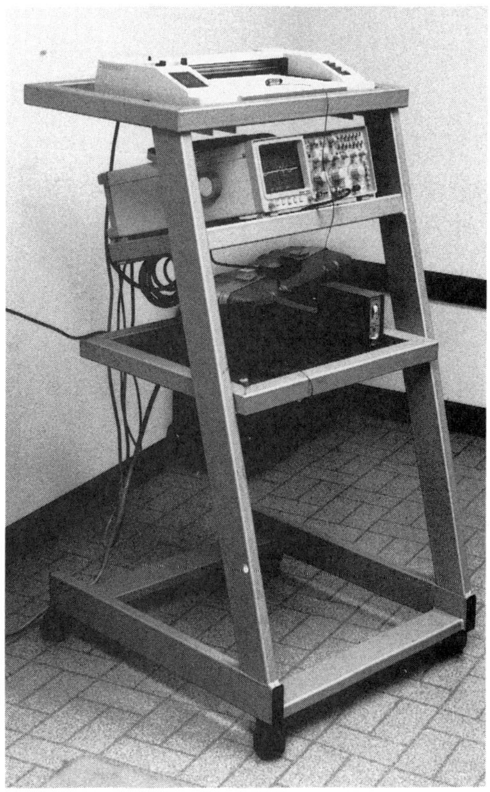

B

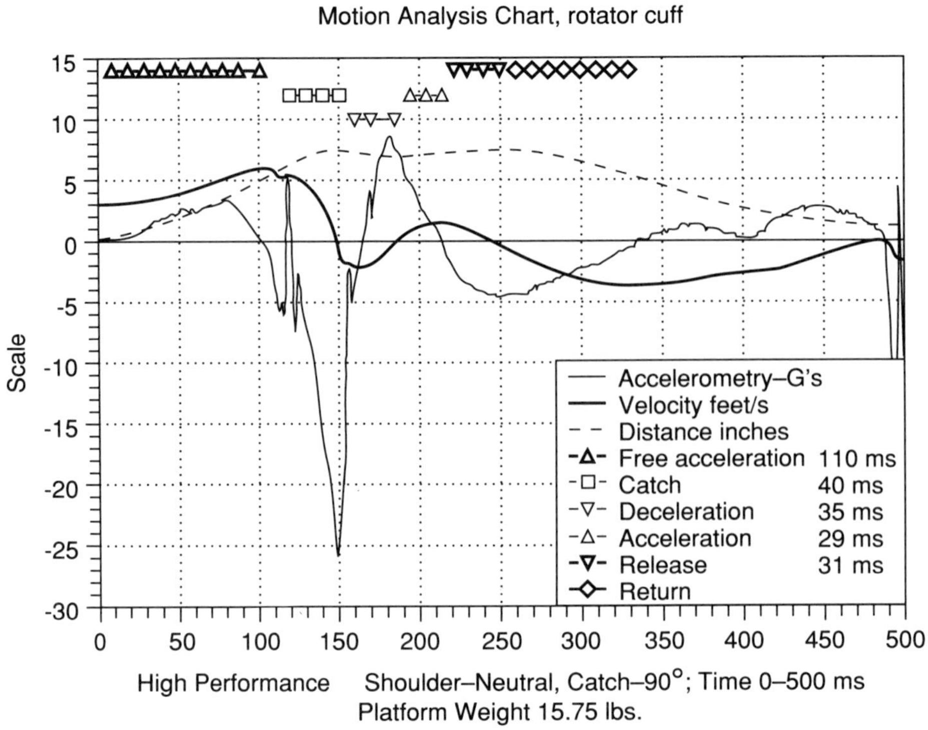

Fig. 5-6. Single repetition accelerometry force curve (units express in Gs). Peak acceleration above baseline; eccentric output below baseline; accelerometer calibrated for 10 millivolts = 1 G.

lected accelerometry to investigate force-velocity relationships, while Grabiner[18] used accelerometry to study the effects of electromechanical delay on the SEC. Although there is limited information on reliability/validity issues,[19,20] accelerometry provides a means of clinical documentation and patient assessment, performance testing, and perhaps most importantly at this early stage in the understanding of inertial exercise, the capability to perform clinical and experimental research.

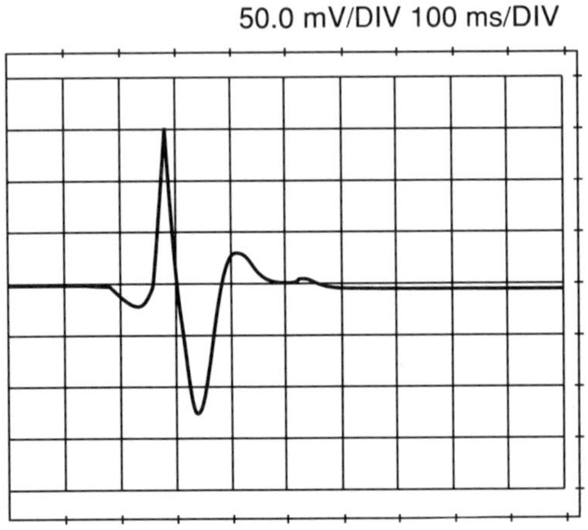

Fig. 5-7. Computerized analysis of accelerometry data (shoulder external rotation movement).

The limited use of a linear piezometric accelerometer package has proved beneficial and educational for patient assessment and description of basic muscular responses and force properties with Impulse applications. The four components of this single axis accelerometer package are as follows (also see Fig. 5-5):

1. Accelerometer: Model 302A PCB-Piezotronics, 3245 Walden Ave., DePew, NY 14043
2. Oscilloscope: Digital Storage Oscilloscope, B&K Precision Co., 6460 West Cortland St., Chicago, IL 60016
3. Plotter: Model SP 600/601 XY Plotter, Enter Computer, Inc., 6867 Nancy Ridge Dr., San Diego, CA 92121

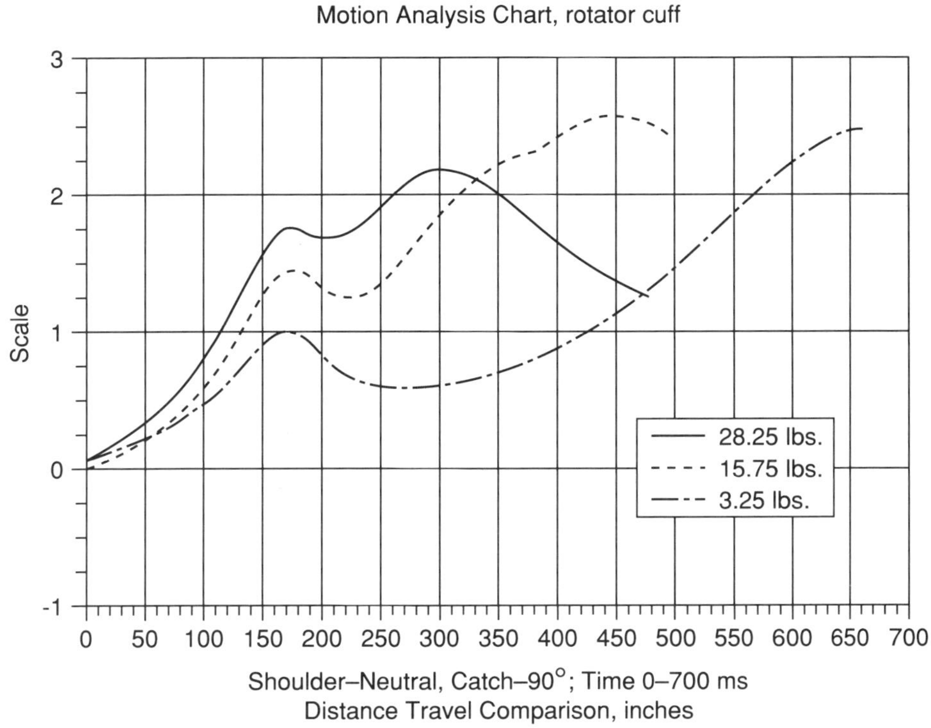

Fig. 5-8. Computerized comparison of travel of platform at three different masses.

4. Interface: EMA, Inc., P.O. Box 2312, Newnan, GA 30326

The concentric/eccentric force responses of a given muscle group, which are recorded on an accelerometry curve by the plotter (Fig. 5-6), form the basis of force measurement and comparison, with the potential for additional analysis and enhancement from computer programs (Figs. 5-7 and 5-8). The accelerometer system is calibrated so that 10 millivolts = 1 G of response.

CLINICAL CONCEPTS OF INERTIAL EXERCISE

Although based on empirical evidence from 3½ years of varied clinical usage, inertial exercise appears to be safe, versatile, and effective with multiple orthopaedic and sports biomechanical movement dysfunctions and injuries. The Impulse inertial unit varies from traditional pulley units in that the eccentric component occurs in a short movement range (less than 10 degrees) and at high velocity. By virtue of Impulse's high frequency rate (defined as repetitions per second) (Thein, unpublished material, 1988) and common use of submaximal resistance, the system functions as a neuromuscular re-education device that supplements traditional strength training techniques.

An operational definition of the type of loading that the Impulse produces is "horizontal, sub-maximal, gravity eliminated plyometrics." The concept of submaximal plyometrics, involving controlled eccentric loads, is an attractive clinical feature as part of a time phased functional progression. During each repetition, tissue elasticity from the eccentric catch is transferred into kinetic energy to potentiate the concentric phase. This occurs without gravitational and frictional loads, and therefore can be applied to both isolated joints early in rehabilitation and to mass movement, kinetic chain activities during more advanced phases of

Table 5-1. Hip Extension Eccentric Versus Concentric Force Ratios at Varying Masses (on Platform)

Weight (lb)	Eccentric (G)	Concentric (G)	Ratio[a]
25	30.0	7.5	4
20	25.5	9.45	2.69
15	18.2	7	2.6
10	25.2	7.7	3.27
5	30.1	11.9	2.53

[a] Ratio = eccentric value/concentric value.

rehabilitation, or to specific performance training programs.

An interesting biomechanical characteristic of inertial loading involves the eccentric/concentric force ratio of a single muscle or group of muscles. As demonstrated in Table 5-1 the eccentric/concentric ratio is at least 1, with increased ratios above 3 corresponding to higher speeds of motion. With inertial loading and accelerometry documentation, a similiar consistent ratio exists. For example, with shoulder external rotation, using 3.25 lb on the sliding platform, the eccentric force produced by one male subject was 403 ft-lb and concentric force was 135 ft-lb yielding a 2.99 ratio. A similiar relationship can be demonstrated in the lower extremity (Table 5-2).

Special Clinical Considerations

In traditional isotonic resistive exercise conditions, as the load is increased there is increased stress applied to the system in a concept called overload. This principle of adaptation of body tissues to increased demands forms the basis for many training regimens and is organized into specific programs known as progressive resistive exercise (PRE). A primary contrasting feature of inertial exercise with other resistive modes is the unique reversal of the relationship between the amount of resistance load and the increased stress applied to the musculoskeletal system. Inertial exercise behaves in an opposite manner, which can be called regressive resistive exercise (RRE). With inertial loading, when the mass (weight applied to the sliding platform) is high, inherent inertial properties lower the acceleration (resultant force) and deceleration. It is clear that initial acceleration is dependent on concentric muscular contraction, which has a definite peak threshold. As training advances or rehabilitation progresses, greater stress is applied to the tissue by using a lower weight; this in turn corresponds to higher speed of the sliding platform and working joint. As speed increases, both concentric and eccentric force output increase, with a larger percentage change in the eccentric component. This relationship has been consistently verified with the use of accelerometry study for varied joint and involved muscle groups (Table 5-2). As demonstrated in Table 5-2, it appears that many individuals perform best with inertial loading within a narrow range of working mass. This so-called "power zone" is highly individual and variable but probably relates to a specific neuromuscular control mechanism. As exceedingly high weights are used, the force potentials decrease by an unexplained yet, perhaps, protective mechanism. Consequently, inertial loading produces an alteration in both the force-velocity curve and the standard concept of overload progression. One important note about eccentric force during high speed movements relates to the possibility that this eccentric catch is performed in a proportionately long period of time relative to the concentric phase, resulting in

Table 5-2. Upper Extremity Forces and Speed at Various Loads

Mass (lb)	Average Deceleration (G)	Average Acceleration (G)	Deceleration (msec)	Acceleration (msec)	Power (ft-lb/sec)
3.25	4	1	38	46	.5
15.75	14.2	8.75	46	55	4.4
28.25	6.06	2.32	112	240	.5

(Performed with standing shoulder external rotation, arm adducted to netural, elbow flexed to 90°.)

a dissipation effect that may be an important safety feature. During high speed movements with the Impulse system, both the concentric and eccentric phases occur in less than 100 milliseconds. Such a dissipation of eccentric force is speculative and, of course, needs additional investigation. Another differential event of Impulse loading compared with other resistive modes of exercise, involves the use of a small training arc of motion (often 30 degrees or less) that is reduced as the velocity or frequency rate of the exercise increases. The potential disadvantage of limited arc motion, coupled with high speed, is loss of joint stability. However, it appears that appropriate progression of inertial training produces an adaptation that supersedes any biomechanical deficiency.

The location and alignment of working axes represent the final unique difference between Impulse and other types of resistive apparatus. The Impulse operates through a series of three distinct pulleys (one of which is adjustable), which function together as a unit. This pulley unit is then interfaced to the human's working joint in a three-dimensional position. The working axis is a complex interaction of multiple planes of movement and may exist at a point outside of the patient's body and in an oblique angle to the working joint. This concept can be initially frustrating for the patient and health care professional to visualize, select, and control. The selection of the optimal working axis is quickly learned by combining the appropriate position of the pulley that is mounted to the vertical post with the appropriate position of patient relative to the Impulse unit. Body position variations between patients for the same exercise pattern can be pronounced due to individual skeletal lever lengths and the associated vectors of force.

Clinical Timing and Progression

As with other types of resistive apparatus or rehabilitation techniques, optimal results and safety principles depend on appropriate timing and correct progression. Two key terms applied to the clinical effects of inertial exercise are *tonic* and *phasic* training. Tonic training involves a constant tension on the resistance line during transitions from concentric to eccentric muscle loading and refers to optimal joint stability. In contrast, phasic training involves higher speeds and lighter mass on the platform, and alternating periods of line tension and slack that function to recruit dynamic joint stability. Phasic types of inertial training produce cyclic bursts of muscular cocontractions across a given working joint. In addition, early inertial training uses single joint axes, with isolated muscles prior to mass patterns.

Table 5-3. Davies Exercise Progression Continuum

Multiple angle isometrics (submaximal effort)
Multiple angle isometrics (maximal), inertial
Short arc concentric isokinetics (submaximal), inertial
Short arc isotonics
Short arc concentric isokinetics (maximal)
Full ROM concentric isokinetics (submaximal)
Full ROM isotonics
Full ROM concentric isokinetics (maximal)

(Adapted from Davies,[21] with permission.)

A useful clinical progression scheme is reviewed in Table 5-3, which is adapted from Davies[21] and integrates other common forms of muscle training. As a general rule, after injuries or dysfunction, inertial loading should progress from heavy mass to lighter mass, and from tonic applications to more phasic protocols (Fig. 5-9). The following primary techniques for inertial training are taken from Davison, personal correspondence, 1989.

Phasic programs

1. Slack protocol with catch waiting: the subject pulls the line through the range of motion

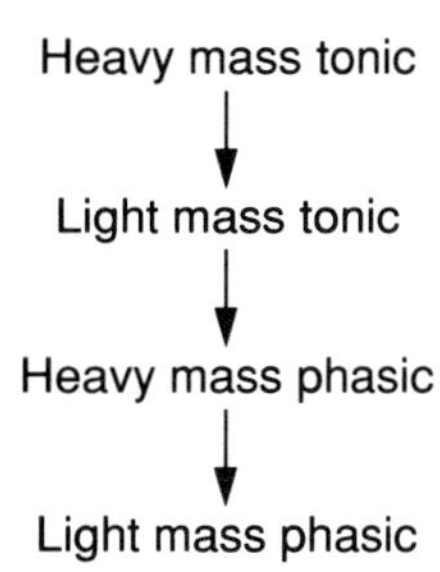

Fig. 5-9. Phased progression of Impulse for increased stress.

(ROM) from the IP to the FP (Fig. 5-3), accelerating the platform mass. At FP the subject quickly returns to the IP, producing a momentary slack in the line that allows the platform to coast along the track. At IP, the subject waits for the line to tighten, which creates a slight jerk, and catches the momentum of the mass and brings it to a sudden halt. (This is generally an intermediate or advanced program.

2. Slack protocol with catch anticipation: the subject pulls the line through the ROM from IP to FP, accelerating the platform. At FP the subject quickly returns to the IP, which produces a slack in the line, and allows the platform to coast along the track. At IP the subject anticipates the catch phase, accelerating the limb to meet the momentum of the platform. This anticipation creates an instantaneous halting of the platform while simultaneously accelerating the platform into the next repetition. This is an intermediate or advanced program, although people with good coordination may master this level earlier.

Tonic programs

3. No slack protocol: the subject pulls the line through the ROM from IP to FP, accelerating the platform in continued effort at the FP. When the subject feels the momentum of the platform pulling on the line he decelerates the platform throughout the return to IP. As IP is reached, a smooth transition of acceleration to deceleration is produced. This level is recommended for beginning training.

Based on clinical results from over 500 patient/athlete training sessions, the indications for inertial training are numerous and diverse (Table 5-4). As clinical usage grows and research results are integrated into clinical programs, the breadth and type of indications will surely undergo transitions. The speculative issues of inertial training effects on bone mass and strength (described in the section *Proposed Inertial Loading*), capsular afference, and physiologic overflow to the contralateral side all possess tremendous potential for future applications. Capsular afference and feedback or proprioceptive loops have been demonstrated in animal models[22] and in several recent studies regarding human knee arthrology.[23–25]

Table 5-4. Application for Inertial Training

Conditions
Submaximal plyometrics
Neuromuscular training
Training of tendon tissue
Alteration of electromechanical delay
Physiologic crossover effects
Indications
Painful arc remediation
Mechanical, reproducible joint pain
Capsular afference/coordination
Proposed prevention of bone loss

The pilot study, presented in the section *Research and Case Studies*, demonstrates statistical evidence for a crossover effect on the contralateral, untrained side.

With athletes, training can often advance rapidly without specific program structure as explained above with the simple guiding principle of reducing the mass as quickly as the athlete can gain control and simultaneously attempting to achieve the highest frequency rate possible (with some motions as fast as 4 repetitions per second). In nonathletes or in cases where soft tissue healing constraints or joint arthrokinematic problems are paramount, progress may be best served by reducing the mass in 2.5-lb decrements. The chief consideration is use of a mass that enables the subject to work with control of the particular movement pattern and protocol objective. In cases where coordination is poor, increasing the mass will assist in proper control. Impulse training is safely initiated in the subacute period after injury or flare-up of chronic joint conditions.

Guidelines for starting inertial training include a conservative allowance for restoration of 75 percent of active ROM that is available in a given plane of motion and the control of pain in a joint or soft tissues that is caused by movement. Due to the intolerance of articular cartilage to instantaneous peak loads (impulses), precautions must be taken when introducing inertial training after prolonged immobilization, which can soften and decrease the stiffness of articular cartilage. An indirect sign of articular cartilage strain is the onset of joint effusion; this is also a relative contraindication for inertial training.

Despite the fact that innate motor control may vary significantly between the upper limbs, lower

Table 5-5. Suggested Starting Weights with Inertial Exercise

Upper extremity
Shoulder: male, 17.5–10 lb; female, 15–10 lb
Elbow: male, 17.5–10 lb; female, 15–10 lb
Wrist: male, 10 lb; female, 7.5–5 lb
Lower extremity
Hip: male, 30–20 lb; female, 20–15 lb
Knee: male, 30–20 lb; female, 20–15 lb
Ankle: male, 15–10 lb; female, 10–7.5 lb
Trunk
Lumbar rotation, 30–25 lb
Cervical flexion, 15 lb

Mass selected on the basis of relative body weight and limb segment weight.

limbs, and spine within a single subject, it is important to have a guideline for the correct mass in the initial training session. A suggested starting weight for various body parts and motions is outlined in Table 5-5 (Thein, unpublished material, 1988). Weights selected should always produce comfortable training bouts and fatigue, without residual joint or muscle pain. Although it is unexplained, even intense training with inertial loads has not resulted in a single reported case of delayed onset muscle soreness (DOMS) in the audit of over 500 patient/athlete cases.

The final principle for an effective inertial exercise program design involves the structure of a single session of Impulse IES training. In 1986, secondary to 1 year of clinical usage, a general approach to mixed sports and orthopaedic dysfunction was developed and designated as *Albert's Rule of Threes* (Table 5-6). The Rule of Threes was designed as a compromise between principles of exercise physiology, soft tissue healing constraints, motor learning theory, and ease in patient/subject orientation and compliance. It enables the patient to work a demanding, specific session in a safe environment with the facilitating effects of muscular fatigue on motor skill acquisition structured in a time efficient manner.

Table 5-6. Albert's Rule of Threes: Single Inertial Exercise Session Design

Three repetitions per second (a fast but controllable speed)
Three work bouts of 30 seconds
Three work sessions per week
Three movement patterns for each specific joint
Thirty second rest periods between bouts

PROPOSED INERTIAL LOADING EFFECTS ON BONE MASS AND REMODELING DYNAMICS*

The muscular and mechanical stresses from regular physical activity promote and maintain adequate bone mineral content (BMC).[26] Individuals engaging in vigorous physical activity demonstrate higher BMC than sedentary people.[27,28] People living in a weightless environment (as seen in space travel) also experience a decrease in both muscle mass and BMC.[29,30]

Bone remodeling increases in anatomic areas where forces are applied.[31,32] For example, the dominant arms of tennis and baseball players demonstrate higher BMC than the nondominant arms. In addition, people who perform explosive or resistive exercises (e.g., weight lifters and sprinters) tend to have higher BMC than people who perform predominately endurance type activities.[33,34]

For purposes of the present discussion, two primary concepts regarding stress and strain will be differentiated. First, mechanical stress is characterized by activities that involve relatively constant forces, with low energy demands that are expended over long periods of time. Primary examples of mechanical stress activity include walking, standing, and distance running. In contrast, dynamic strain activities, such as weight lifting, team sports, and sprinting or jumping, involve high forces with brief onset that require instantaneous elastic stretch to the involved tissues. It appears that exercises that produce dynamic strain are more influential than mechanical stressors in bone remodeling and BMC.[35,36] Inertial exercises, applied through the Impulse system, produces cyclic, vigorous dynamic strain that may positively affect bone remodeling, bone strength, and BMC levels.

* This section was provided by Steve Davison, of Engineering Marketing Associates, Newnan, GA.

Connective Tissue and Motor Unit Behavior Produced by Impulse

Dynamic strain is imposed on bone by connective tissue tension and impact, or impulse, forces from contact with an external object. The karate chop is an example of both types of strain. Active motor units in arm and forearm musculature accelerate the forearm to 200 feet per second in a brief period of less than 250 milliseconds.[37] Immediately prior to contact, the active motor units turn off, with resultant impact forces of 250 ft-lb created by the moment of inertia. Kicking produces a similiar motor activity with summation of kinetic chain forces.[38] Dynamic strain to bone depends on tension from motor units that is applied to tendon.[39] Muscles concentrically contract in ballistic movements (e.g., karate chop), and eccentrically respond to forceful stretch load that is imposed on the skeletal system. In either case, tension and force are generated rapidly, as it is in inertial training. As the speed of muscular contraction increases, the difference between concentric and eccentric forces also increases.[40]

Muscle Fiber Recruitment

Muscle fiber types, classified as type I or type II, demonstrate different functional recruitment patterns. Type I is recruited for tonic or postural activities, while type II is recruited for short, intense performance.[41–44] Type II fibers produce the higher forces and appear to function selectively in preprogrammed motor activities or in eccentric loading. As described by Seliger et al.,[45] eccentric motor activities produce two to three times the force of concentric activities. Consequently, conscious motor control of a specific activity will slow down resulting movement due to the recruitment of type I fiber.[43] Although all muscle fibers tend to be activated in any given movement, there exists a fiber recruitment order and selective hierarchy as presented in Fig. 5-10.

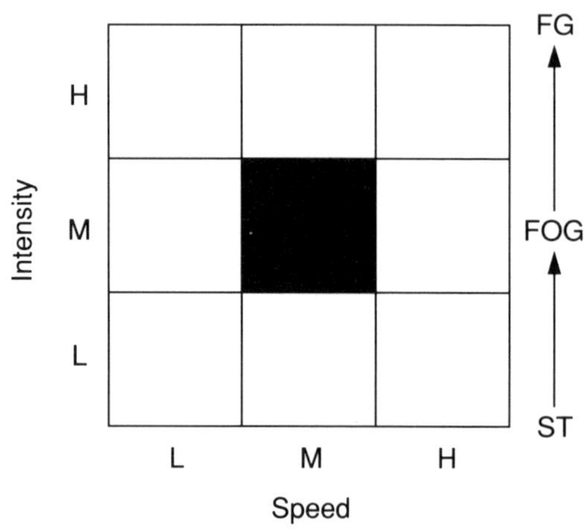

Fig. 5-10. Fiber type recruitment order. L, low; M, medium; H, high.

Gravity Considerations on Bone Mass/Remodeling

BMC is increased in response to increased load on the lower limb, regardless of gravitational effects. It has been demonstrated that activities performed in an essentially gravity-free setting such as baseball pitching, hitting a tennis ball, or kicking a soccer ball all produce increased BMC.[28] In addition, high compressive joint forces can be produced by high tension levels from tendons.[38] The Impulse unit, which is designed to operate in a gravity-free environment, has the potential to influence BMC and to create bone remodeling through its dynamic strain type of exercise.

Conclusions

The Impulse produces high velocity tendon tension and recruits type II fibers with high speed eccentric demands. In order to optimize inertial loading effects on bone mineral status, the Impulse would be best applied to multiple body areas with use of isolated muscle groups as well as total kinetic chain applications.

Inertial exercise performed on both muscular and connective tissues has the potential to prevent loss of bone mass or reverse osteopenia in individuals living in weightless environments (such as bedrest/immobilized patients and astronauts in prolonged space travel), and in people with signs of osteoporosis. Extensive research on the interaction of inertial loading and bone strength, mass, and architecture is indicated, with many interesting and important future applications.

RESEARCH PERSPECTIVES AND CASE STUDIES WITH IMPULSE

As with any new product, clinical usage and development and completion of research studies progress gradually. An overview of some available studies are presented in this section with several clinical case studies and an appendix listing abstracts that refer to inertial exercise research or use. The emphasis of this section is on the potential for continued investigation and the identification of several worthy questions or designs for future research efforts. Indeed, the state of the art with inertial exercise is at an early stage in scientific verification and discovery.

Inertial Exercise Pilot Study

Performed in 1987, the following study was designed to investigate the training effects of inertial loading on upper extremity muscle (biceps brachii) in normal subjects, as related to the possibility that one phase of an inertial exercise repetition was isokinetic. The null hypothesis was that inertial training does not produce significant high speed isokinetic torque increases in biceps brachii of normal human subjects.

Methods

With informed consent as approved by an institutional review board, 33 subjects were selected by a screening questionnaire that identified previous history of any cervical/bilateral upper extremity trauma and routine patterns of recreational or competitive use of either upper extremity. all customary upper extremity activities were continued unchanged and no new activities were permitted during the study period. Three subjects were deleted from the study, one due to mild shoulder capsular injury of undetermined cause and the others due to failure to comply with the requirement of completion of a minimum of 12 training sessions in the 5-week training period.

The dominant hand was determined per subject as the preferred hand for writing or throwing movements, with 26 of the 30 subjects who completed the study being right handed. Each subject served as their own control with only the nondominant side receiving the 5-week training program. Subject demographics are outlined in Table 5-7. Subjects were pretested on a Lido Digital Isokinetic system (Loredon Biomedical, Inc., Davis, CA) and post-tested within 1 week of completing the training sessions. Testing was performed in supine position (Fig. 5-11) using elbow flexion/extension at 90 degrees per second and 300 degrees per second with three maximal efforts at each speed following 5-warmup repetitions at 120 degrees per second and supine manual stretch to biceps brachii muscle for a 1 minute static hold (Fig. 5-12).

Experimental design ensured that trunk and shoulder position were maintained identically in both training and testing setups. The trunk was maintained in neutral extension/rotation, while the glenohumeral joint was fixed in neutral flexion/extension and the humerus was fully adducted and maintained in neutral rotation. Scapular stabilization was maintained through body weight compression against the supporting surface (respectively, the chair back in training and the Lido table in testing. Throughout the study, the pulley position on the Impulse vertical post was fixed at 8 inches from the floor. The straight back chair

Table 5-7. Subject Demographics (Mean ± SD)

Variable	Males (N = 10)	Females (N = 20)	Total (N = 30)
Age (yr)	23.8 ±3.4	22.0 ± 2.3	22.6 ± 2.9
Weight (lb)	177.9 ± 34.2	123.7 ± 12.6	141.5 ± 34

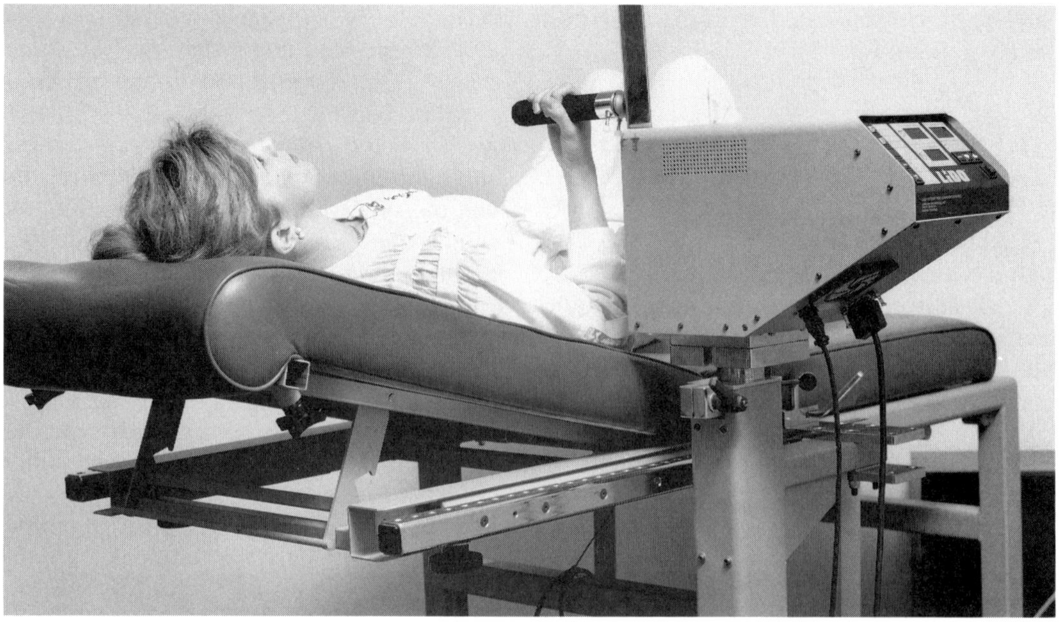

Fig. 5-11. Pilot study, testing position.

used for training sessions was positioned so that each subject's individual trunk and limb length, relative to the fixed axis, allowed smooth control between the concentric and eccentric responses of the elbow flexors (Fig. 5-13). Prior to training, each subject was thoroughly oriented to required protocol, basic operation of the Impulse unit, and specific movement task of coordinated reversal of the weight platform. Finally, subjects were allowed supervised trial training periods of 5 minutes on the Impulse. No method was devised to quantify the subject's effort level, other than concise instructions to pull as hard as possible and to reverse the weight platform as fast as possible, in order to maximize the repetitions per 30-second work bout.

Based on the clinical protocol (Rule of Threes) described in Table 5-6, training sessions were performed a minimum of twice weekly and a maximum of 3 times weekly with at least 1 day between each session. Each session was immediately preceded with the manual stretch previously described. Training sessions were structured with a partner system, in which the training person was seated, stabilized, and commanded to go and stop by the supervising partner, who then simultaneously timed the bout with a stopwatch and visually monitored the appropriate speed and platform excursion (Table 5-8).

Experimental data analysis was used to detect a significant interaction of arm (trained versus control) and session (pre- versus post-test), with an increse in high speed isokinetic force predicted in the trained arm from pre- to post-test and no increase in the control arm from pre- to post-test. All torque values generated during testing were recorded directly from IBM microcomputer calculations of force, which for Lido system software and dynamometer is instantaneously and continuously self-calibrated. Computation of statistical means and associated tests of Repeated Measures of analysis of variance (ANOVA) were performed using the CLR ANOVA package by McIntosh.

Results

Both intrasubject and intersubject torque values (Table 5-9) demonstrated large variability that appears to be a function of individual neuromuscular factors and is unrelated to body weight/torque ratios. Such ratios are determined by dividing the

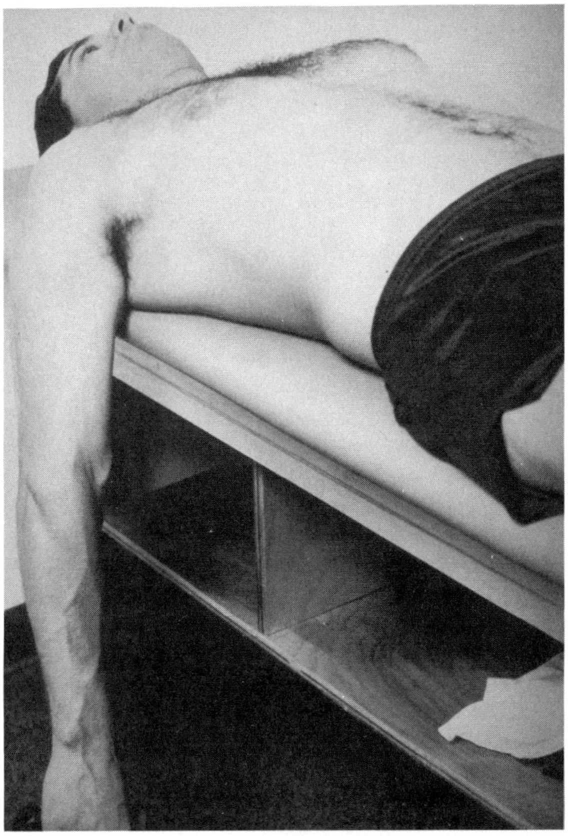

Fig. 5-12. Static stretch position for long head of biceps tendon. Wrist is pronated with internally rotated shoulder.

body weight in pounds into peak torque expressed in foot-pounds.

Twelve of the 30 subjects (11 of which were females) produced no torque changes from pre to post-test. Also, in 3 of the 60 total isokinetic tests performed, subjects were unable to register torque on any of three successive maximal efforts at the set speeds. Although a small torque increase of means from pre to post-test groups (1.2 ft-lb) occurred at 300 degrees per second, the change should be considered with respect to the extreme coefficients of variation, 83.3 percent and 78.6 percent for post-test. At both test speeds, the means of all groups increased from pre- to post-test (Table 5-10), although the percentage change was slightly greater for the high speed control group, 2.9 percent. Examination of the four left handed subjects did not indicate any statistical variation from the other subjects.

The Two-Way Repeated Measures ANOVA did not confirm the prediction of an interaction between arm (trained versus control) and session (pre- versus post-test), nor was there a significant effect for the arm. Instead, there was a significant increase in torque from pre- to post-test irrespective of whether the arm was trained or not. The 90 degree per second condition ($f = 5.214$) proved significant at the $P < .05$ level; while the 300 degree per second condition ($f = 7.67$) was significant at the $P < .01$ level. The results support rejection of the null hypothesis. Nonetheless, the magnitude of this biceps brachii muscular torque increase was small with respect to the 5 week training period.

Discussion

Several important factors may have contributed to the clinically small increase of isokinetic torque. As demonstrated by Davies,[21] physiologic overflow occurs at or below training speeds with the primary effects extending only 30 degrees per second intervals. The training protocol used in this study may have occurred at joint speeds well in

Table 5-8. Inertial Training Protocol

Week	Mass (lb)	Tracking Distance (in)	Work Bout (s = seconds)
1	17	24	30 s (×3) and 30 s rest
2	15	24	30 s (×3) and 30 s rest
3	10	24	30 s (×3) and 30 s rest
4	5	20	30 s (×3) and 30 s rest
5	0	20	30 s (×3) and 30 s rest

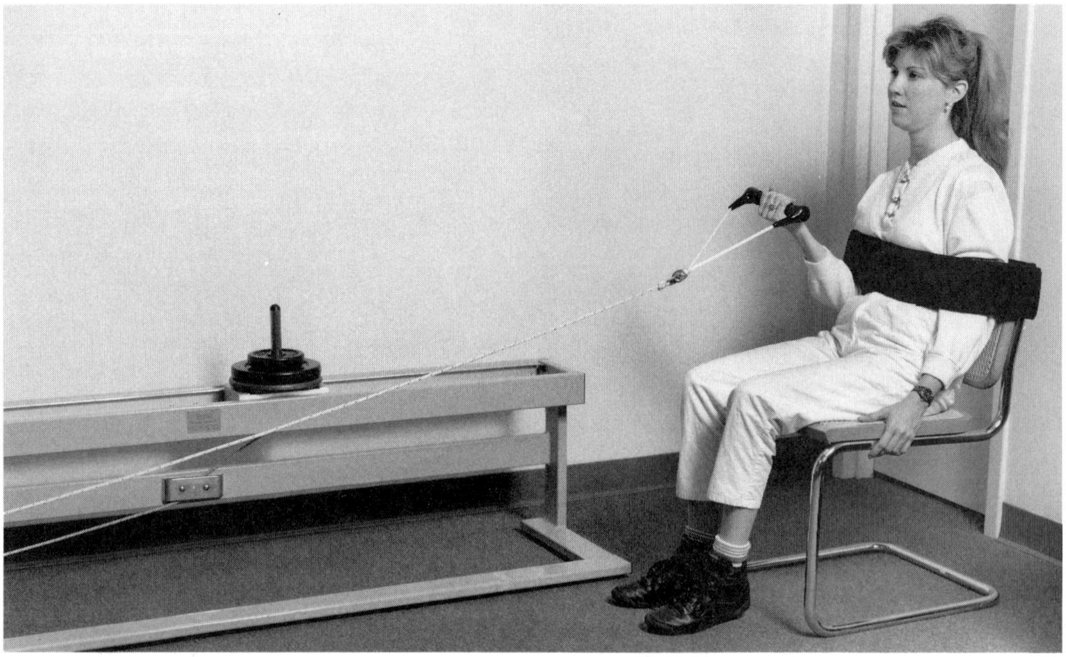

Fig. 5-13. Pilot study, training position.

excess of the test speed examined (300 degrees per second), such that specificity of training effects were negligible. In this study, we made no attempt to calculate the joint speeds reached during training.

Additionally, the subject's degree of volitional effort during the training sessions may have influenced the results. Admittedly, the degree of effort and motivational levels were variable and individual; moreover, the training task of consistently stopping the weight platform on a given reference mark may have produced only submaximal muscular responses that emphasized neuromuscular coordination and cocontraction control at the expense of sufficient overload to produce increased torque.

Other principles characteristic of the Impulse may have influenced the isokinetic test results. First, as speed of the weight platform increases, corresponding to greater demand for stopping and reversing the platform motion, the excursion decreases proportionately. Although testing required approximately 120 degrees of elbow flexion, the training during weeks 3 to 5 only demanded approximately 25 to 30 degrees of active motion. This difference probably contributed to a significant loss of specificity in training results. Second, our testing addressed only concentric effects of the agonist, which neglected to assess the important phase of eccentric loading in inertial exercise as well as the potential changes in the antagonist muscle group. Finally, Rothstein[46] claims that the potential for statistical variation that may have been produced by the Lido's interval scaled measurement responses. It is possible that any or all of these factors may have minimized the degree of torque increases that could result.

A concluding point involves the post-training torque increases of the control extremity. Potential clinical applications, such as use for the contralateral correlate of an immobilized limb, warrant further investigation of the neuromuscular effects on the opposite side of the body. Although speculative in nature, the use of Impulse cross-training benefits provides exciting future use patterns of inertial loads.

Table 5-9. Raw Test Results

	Control-Right		Trained-Left	
Subjects	Pretest	Post-Test	Pretest	Post-Test
1 M	41	57	46	45
2 M	21	14	19	19
3 F	5	14	6	6
4 F	6	7	7	8
5 F	6	5	6	7
6 M	12	13	11	13
7 F	6	6	5	6
8 F	7	6	7	6
9 F	7	9	8	7
10 F	6	7	5	7
11 F	9	9	7	6
12 F	6	7	7	7
13 F	6	5	5	7
14 M	13	13	14	17
15 M	12	10	8	16
16 M	24	31	27	36
17 F	6	6	7	9
18 F	5	5	6	6
19 F	0	6	7	6
20 F	0	7	0	6
21 M	12	17	10	10
22 F	5	7	8	8
23 M	18	14	18	15
24 F	8	7	7	7
25 F	7	7	7	6
26 M	15	14	18	19
27 F	5	6	6	7
28 M	10	11	10	13
29 F	6	7	6	8
30 F	9	9	9	10

Speed = 300 degrees per second; values are expressed in foot-pounds.

Conclusions

1. The Impulse provides a new form of therapeutic and performance exercise with promising applications in musculo-skeletal and neuromuscular disciplines.
2. Inertial exercise, as applied with the Impulse, produces high speed isokinetic torque improvements of the biceps brachii muscle in normal subjects at the .01 level of significance.
3. The complex and novel characteristics of inertial exercise warrant continued clinical investigation and experimental research on many questions: concepts of functional eccentric control; crosstraining effects; optimal clinical program features; reliability/validity testing; and the role in bone mass maintenance.
4. Versatile clinical protocols can be safely applied in time efficient manner with minimal requirements for trainer/therapist supervision.

CASE STUDIES

Case 1

Patient Description: Thirty-four-year-old white man employed as a professional baseball pitcher. Primarily a reliever, the right handed player was a former recipient of the Cy Young Award and is known for his split finger fastball. Due to his physical status, the player is on extended disability from baseball.

Admitting Diagnosis: The patient's current diagnosis was denervated right infraspinatus muscle from suprascapular nerve neuritis with status post-surgical nerve decompression. The patient's complaints were sharp pain when pitching baseball in follow-through phase, dull, aching sensation at rest, extreme weakness with all elevation movements, and need to protect right arm during simple activities of daily living.

Contributory History: Two years of chronic dysfunction with his right shoulder from pitching with history of arthroscopy for debridement and

Table 5-10. Torque Changes (Mean ± SD)

	Control		Trained	
Speed	Pretest	Post-Test	Pretest	Post-Test
90°/s	21.00 (13.06)	22.33 (13.74)	21.43 (12.58)	22.73 (13.15)
300°/s	9.77 (7.98)	11.20 (10.12)	10.23 (8.61)	11.43 (8.97)

acromioplasty of the right acromioclavicular complex, arthrotomy for rotator cuff partial tear repair, and repair of the anterior-superior rim of the glenoid labrum. Upon initial presentation in the clinic, the patient had been unable to pitch for 6 months.

Physical Examination Results: During initial greeting, it was observed that the patient was unable to offer a firm or sustained handshake, due to patient report of weakness and apprehension. Manual muscle tests revealed weakness as follows:

Flexion and abduction, grade 5 –
Supraspinatus isolation, grade 4 –
Internal rotation, grade 4
External rotation, grade 4 –
Infraspinatus trapezius/rhomboids, grade 4 –

Active ROM was normal with exception of internal rotation, restricted to 50 degrees (at 90 abducted position), compared with 80 of left shoulder. A pronounced loss of scapular control with winging was observed in eccentric flexion at 80 degrees until 20 degrees. Cervical rotation was restricted to right as compared with left, 65/80 degrees, while cervical overpressure, compression, and distraction were all nonpainful. Tenderness was noted in the supraspinatus, long-head of biceps, greater tuberosity of humerus and C-5,6 interspace. Soft tissue tightness was noted in the pectoralis major, subscapularis, and supraspinatus. In addition, pronounced atrophy was noted in the pectoralis major, upper trapezius, deltoid, and infraspinatus. Grip strength was reduced by 10 kilograms on the right, with three maximal efforts summated into one value.

Program Structure: The entire program was instituted on a 3 times per week basis over a 37 week period, during which the patient missed a total of 3 weeks for personal reasons.

Electrical stimulation of functional type as well as direct current stimulation were used to stimulate the suprascapular nerve. Although dysfunction of the suprascapular nerve is infrequently reported in young athletes, it is apparently a common occurrence, but is often missed as a diagnosis in many throwing athletes and those who use forceful, overhead motions.[47,48] The electrical stimulation was discontinued due to minimal patient response after 3 weeks. The following multimodal exercise program served as the primary therapeutic modality:

Home program of isotonics with free weights and machines as indicated, and isodynamics in specific patterns/positions
Manual and proprioceptive neuromuscular facilitation (PNF) resistance
Isokinetics with velocity spectrum training, progressing from plane of the scapula external/internal rotation to straight plane flexion and finally to PNF D2 patterns
Impulse inertial training beginning in the fourth week of rehabilitation, preceded by testing on accelerometer (Table 5-11), with multiple patterns performed in the standing position for specificity to throwing demands, the patterns progressing from internal rotation to external rotation and finally to overhead throwing like motions to simulate high speed, eccentric loads encountered in pitching.
After 30 weeks of rehabilitation, a graduated, supervised and symptom-guided toss-throw progression with full speed pitching as the final goal
Specific warmdown stretches and cryotherapy administered after each clinical session and each throwing period

Program Results: Final assessments were performed in the 35th week, with an additional 2 weeks of follow-up and consultation on throwing progressions and in-season weight and mainte-

Table 5-11. Case Study Test Results[a]

	Pretest	Post-Test	% Change
Concentric	.8	7.5	938
Eccentric	1	10.05	1,005

[a] Standing external rotation with 20° abducted position, elbow flexed to 90°. Units expressed in G; 20-lb mass.

nance program design. Prior to discharge the patient status was as follows:

Full, painfree ROM of cervical and glenohumer-joints
Fully controlled scapulohumeral mechanics.
All manual muscle tests grade 5, with exception of external rotation, grade 4+, and abduction, grade 5−.
Resolution of soft tissue tightness and trigger points
Isokinetic strength in PNF diagonals; right, 10 percent stronger than left in flexion-abduction at slow speed and 40 percent stronger at 300 degrees per second.
Inertial testing demonstrated tremendous gains in eccentric and concentric acceleration forces (Table 5-11). The bilateral force curves of external rotation were highly consistent in shape and magnitude in the final inertial testing (Figs. 5-14 and 5-15).
Pitching off the mound with normal body mechanics and peak ball speeds of 90 miles per hour and greater.
No pain at rest or during or after pitching.

Case 2

Patient Description: Twenty-eight-year-old-black man in excellent health, well muscled, and employed as stock clerk in a warehouse.

Admitting Diagnosis and Chief Complaint: The patient's diagnosis was partial rotator cuff tear of left shoulder. The patient described injuring the left shoulder (right hand dominant) during pulling and lowering a heavy box (50 to 80 lb) from an overhead rack. The patient experienced immediate sharp pain, but was able to complete the shift. During that evening and throughout the next day the patient experienced increased left shoulder pain of a deep, constant nature, and weakness. The patient's chief complaint upon presentation in the clinic 8 days postinjury was sharp pain and

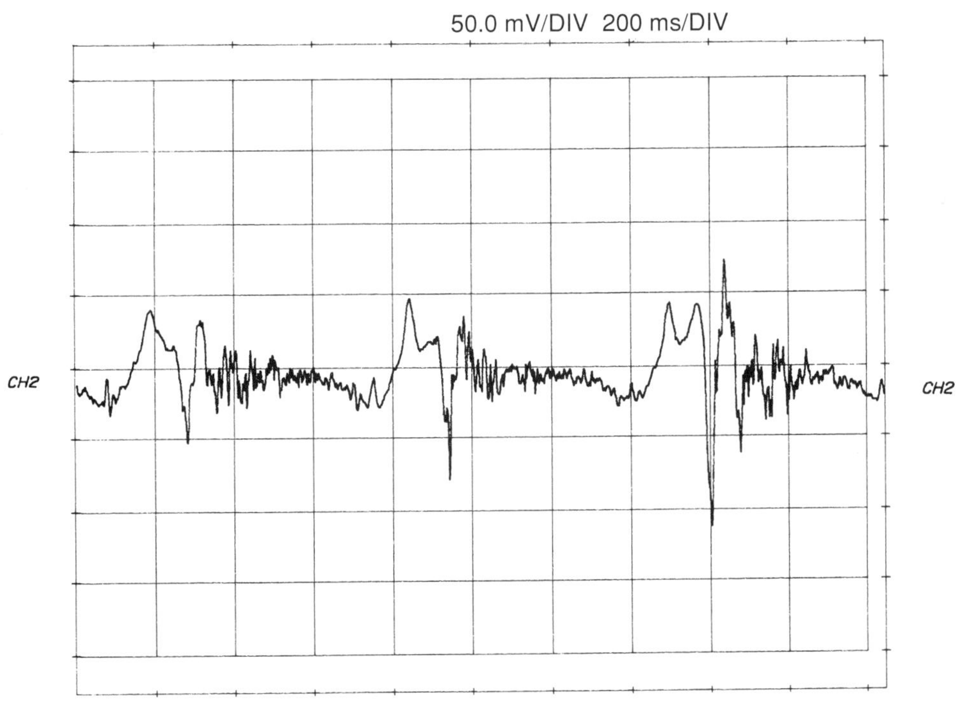

Fig. 5-14. Accelerometry raw curve of patient's external rotation of left nonpitching shoulder.

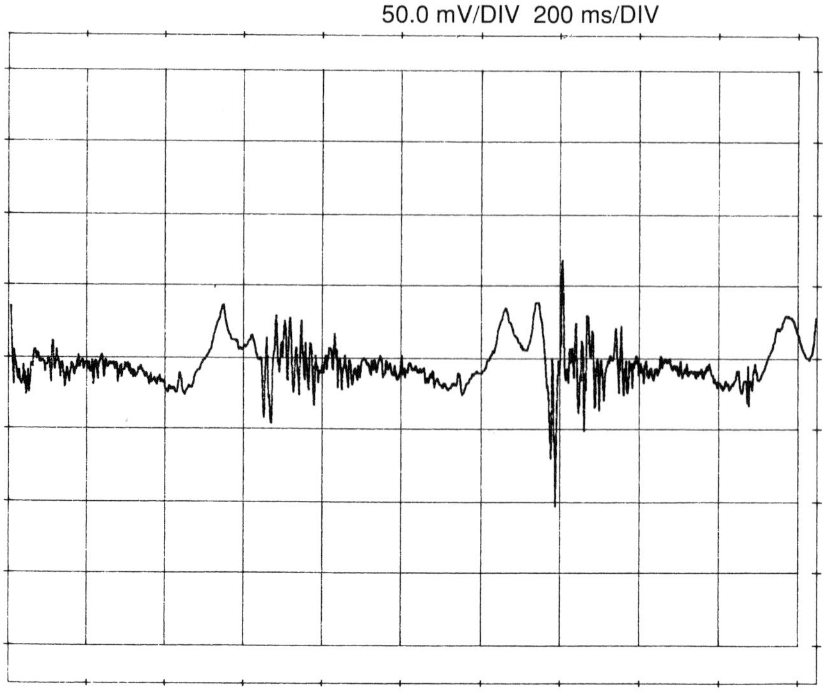

Fig. 5-15. Accelerometry raw curve of patient's external rotation of right shoulder, injured side.

episodic "popping" in selected positions and ROM. The patient denied previous left shoulder dysfunction.

Contributory History: Not applicable.

Physical Examination Results: Global pain of level 6 was reported in specific positions. According to Maitland,[49] the patient demonstrated P1 in shoulder flexion at 125 degrees and P2 at 165 degrees.

Manual muscle tests (right/left = R/L) revealed the following:

Flexion and abduction, R/L, 5/5 –
Supraspinatus isolation, R/L, 5/5
External rotation, R/L, 5/4
Internal rotation, R/L, 5/4

The patient demonstrated joint crepitus of glenohumeral joint palpable as a "click" at 60 degrees of external rotation (actively, supine). External rotation (at 90 degrees of abduction) was restricted to 78 degrees.

Patient demonstrated diffuse tenderness of greater tuberosity with all special tests demonstrating negative results.

Impression: The patient demonstrated a mild rotator cuff tendonitis/partial tear with possible labrum dysfunction and mild impingement presentation.

Program Structure: The patient was instructed in a 5-phase, light load, high repetition isotonic exercise program for home use on a 2 times per day basis and the use of cryotherapy postexercise or during pain periods. The patient was seen in the clinic for an Impulse inertial program as follows:

Day 1, 17 ½-lb resistance load, 3 bouts of 30 seconds each with 3 patterns in the standing position: internal and external rotation with elbow fixed in 90 degree flexed position and shoulder in 20 degrees of abduction, and standing shoulder flexion from a starting point of 15 degrees of hyperextension with slight elbow flexion and fully supinated wrist

Day 2, same program as above with decrease to 15 lb

Day 3, same program

Day 4, same program with weight decrease to 12 ½ lb

Program Results: After the first Impulse session, the patient reported a pain level of 0, with P1 and P2 both at 170 degrees, limited by a sensation of stiffness. After the second session the patient demonstrated manual muscle test grade 5 for all motions except external rotation, grade 4+, with active supine external rotation restricted at 80 degrees by "pop." At the third session the patient demonstrated grade 5 shoulder external rotation, global pain level 0, and active external rotation to 90 degrees, with persistent "pop" at 80 degrees. At the fourth session the patient demonstrated bilateral equal external/internal rotation torque isokinetically (tested on Lido supine at 45 degrees of abduction). The patient discharged himself after this visit and was lost for further follow-up.

Case 3

Patient Description: A twenty-seven-year-old woman in excellent general health, employed in sedentary office position with no regular physical activity.

Admitting Diagnosis and Chief Complaint: The patient was seen with a diagnosis of capsular laxity of the left shoulder. The patient described a gradual onset of pain caused by lifting arm overhead over a 6-month period. The chief complaint was sharp pain at specific positions of flexion.

Contributory History: The patient had a history of competitive gymnastics for 7 years with an acquired ability to voluntarily subluxate both shoulders posteriorly. The patient denied any shoulder injuries during gymnastics that caused missed time from the sport.

Physical Examination Results: Global pain of level 5 was reported during elevation movements. Active ROM was as follows:

Flexion, R/L = 185/110 degrees
Abduction, R/L = 180/120 degrees
External rotation (at 90 degrees of abduction), R/L = 120/106 degrees

The demonstrated P1 in shoulder flexion at 110 degrees and P2 at 120 degrees were limited by a sharp, sudden pain.

Manual muscle tests:

Flexion, R/L = 5/5−
Supraspinatus, internal rotation, and external rotation, R/L = 5/4−
Abduction, R/L = 5/4

Bilateral protracted scapulae, with increased upper thoracic kyphosis and ventral fault position of left humeral head were found. Special tests revealed positive impingement and posterior laxity of grade 4− level on left. Palpation demonstrated tenderness in the infraspinatus and supraspinatus tendinous musculotendinous portion.

Impression: A biomechanical pain presentation caused by posterior shoulder instability, rotator cuff inflammation and weakness, and impingement dysfunction in elevated positions.

Program Design: The patient was instructed in a home program of light load, high repetition isotonics in protected positions for shoulder internal and external rotation, horizontal extension, prone external rotation with combined horizontal extension movement, and supraspinatus isolation lifts. The patient was seen for clinical visits on a 3-times-per-week basis for 7 total visits. For 5 serial visits, the patient was treated with ultrasound to the posterolateral shoulder with positioning to expose the cuff tissue in its most superficial level.

After the second visit, the patient was started on

a PRE Impulse program using the same protocol outlined in case 2. The patient started with 15-lb resistance load, which was decreased to 12½ lb on the fourth visit and to 10 lb on the sixth visit.

Program Results: On the second visit, the patient's pain level was 2 with P1 and P2 equal at 145 degrees flexion. On the third visit, the patient demonstrated 0 pain level with flexion to 165 degrees, with limitation perceived as stiffness. External rotation strength was grade 4+ with all other motions at grade 5. On the fourth and fifth visits, the pain level continued at 0; however, active flexion range decreased to 150. After the fourth visit, the patient reported no dysfunction with any elevation movements required during activities of daily living. On the sixth visit the patient demonstrated grade 5− external rotation strength with continued flexion to 165 degrees and passive posterior glide at grade 4−. Due to the patient's general glenohumeral hypermobility and return of painfree daily function, the slight restriction of flexion was accepted as protective and the patient was discharged.

Per telephone follow-up, the patient continued to have painfree function after 6 months and started playing recreational tennis.

REFERENCES

1. Biodex Co: Biodex User Newsletter. Shirley, NY, 1987
2. Stanton P, Purdam C: Hamstring injuries in sprinting—the role of eccentric exercise. J Orthop Sports Phys Ther 10:347, 1989
3. Hinton RY: Isokinetic evaluation of shoulder rotational strength in high school baseball pitchers. Am J Sports Med 16:274, 1988
4. Grillner S: The role of muscle stiffness in meeting the changing postural and locomotor requirements for force development by the ankle extensors. Acta Physiol Scand 86:92, 1972
5. Komi PV: Physiological and biomechanical correlates of muscle function: effects of muscle structure and stretch-shortening cycle on force and speed. Exerc Sports Sci Rev 12:81, 1984
6. Bosco C, Komi PV: Potentiation of the mechanical behavior of the human skeletal muscle through prestretching. Acta Physiol Scand 106:467, 1979
7. Chapman AE, Caldwell GE, Selbie WS: Mechanical output following muscle stretch in forearm supination against inertial loads. J Appl Physiol 59:78, 1985
8. Bober T, Jaskolski E, Nowacki Z: Study of eccentric-concentric contraction of the upper extremity muscles. J Biomech 13:135, 1980
9. Pertuzon E, Bouisset S: Instantaneous force-velocity relationship in human muscle. Med Sports 8:230, 1973
10. Hakkinen K, Komi PV: Effect of different combined concentric and eccentric muscle work regimes on maximal strength development. J Hum Move Studies 7:33, 1981
11. Costill DL, Fink WJ, Habansky AJ: Muscle rehabilitation after knee surgery. Phys Sports Med 5:71, 1971
12. Enoka RM: Neuro-Mechanical Basis of Kinesiology. Human Kinetics Books, Champaign, 1988
13. Balogun JA, Farina NT, Fay E: Energy cost determination using a portable accelerometer. Phys Ther 66:1103, 1986
14. Smith KL: Commentary. Phys Ther 66:1108, 1986
15. Troup JDG, Chapman AE: The strength of the flexor and extensor muscles of the trunk. J Biomech 2:49, 1969
16. Steinrauf LK, Pawlus J: Neuro-muscular testing by accelerometer, abstracted. Med Sci Sports Exerc 18:546, 1986
17. Bergmaier G, Neukomm P: The correlation between static muscular force and speed of movement. Med Sports 8:253, 1973
18. Grabiner MD: Bioelectric characteristics of the electromechanical delay preceding concentric contraction. Med Sci Sports Exerc 18:37, 1986
19. Saris WHM: Habitual physical activity in children: methodology and findings in health and disease. Med Sci Sports Exerc 18:253, 1986
20. Montoye HJ, Taylor HL: Measurement of physical activity in population studies: a review. Hum Biol 56:195, 1984
21. Davies GJ: Compendium of Isokinetics in Clinical Usage. 3rd Ed. S & S Publishers, Onalasksa, WI, 1987
22. Gardner E: Reflex muscular responses to stimulation of articular nerves in cat. Am J Physiol 161:133, 1950
23. Schultz RA, Miller DC, Kerr CS, Micheli L: Mechanoreceptors in human cruciate ligaments. J Bone Joint Surg 66A:1072, 1984

24. Kennedy JC, Alexander IJ, Hayes KC: Nerve supply of the human knee and its functional importance. Am J Sports Med 10:329, 1982
25. Solomonow M, Baratta R, Zhou EE et al: The synergistic action of the anterior cruciate ligament and thigh muscles in maintaining joint stability. Am J Sports Med 15:207, 1987
26. Smith EL, Raab DM: Osteoporosis and physical activity. Acta Med Scand, suppl. 711:S149, 1986
27. Kriska AM, Sandler RB, Cauley JA et al: The assessment of historical physical activity and its relation to adult bone parameters. Am J Epidemiol 127:1053, 1988
28. Huddleston AL, Rockwell D, Kulund DN, Harrison RB: Bone mass in lifetime tennis athletes. JAMA 24:1107, 1980
29. Weldon GD: Disuse osteoporosis: physiological aspects. Calcif Tissue Int, suppl. 36:s146, 1984
30. Mack PB, LaChance PA, Vose GP: Bone demineralization of foot and hand of Gemini-titan IV, V, VII astronauts during orbital flight. Am J Roent 100:503, 1967
31. Aisenbrey JA: Exercise in the prevention and management of osteoporosis. Phys Ther 67:1100, 1987
32. Roesler H: The history of some fundamental concepts in bone biomechanics. J Biomech 20:1025, 1987
33. Nilsson BE, Westlin NE: Bone density in athletes. Clin Orthop 77:179, 1971
34. Ayalon J: Dynamic bone loading exercises for postmenopausal women: effect on the density of the distal radius. Arch Phys Med Rehabil 68:280, 1987
35. Martin AD, Houston CS: Osteoporosis, calcium and physical activity. Can Med Assoc J 136:587, 1987
36. Sandler RB: Muscle strength and skeletal competence: implications for early prophylaxis. Calcif Tissue Int 42:281, 1988
37. Cavanaugh PR, Landa J: Biomechanical analysis of the karate chop. Res Q 47:611, 1976
38. Wahrenberg H, Lindbeck L, Ekholm J: Knee muscular moment, tendon tension force and EMG during a vigorous movement in man. Scand J Rehabil Med 10:100, 1978
39. Tipton CM, Vailis AC, Matthes RD: Experimental studies on the influences of physical activity on ligaments, tendons and joints: a brief review. Acta Med Scand, suppl. 711:S157, 1986
40. Komi PV: Measurement of force-velocity relationship in human muscle under concentric and eccentric contractions. Med Sports 8:225, 1973
41. Karlsson J, Sjodin B, Jacobs I, Kaiser P: Relevance of muscle fibre type to fatigue in short intense and prolonged exercise in man. CIBA 82:59, 1981
42. Nilsson J, Tesch P, Thorstensson A: Fatigue and EMG of repeated fast voluntary contractions in man. Acta Physiol Scand 101:194, 1977
43. Kuo KHM, Clamann HP: Coactivation of synergistic muscles of different fiber types in fast and slow contractions. Am J Phys Med 60:219, 1981
44. Saltin B: Muscle fibre recruitment and metabolism in prolonged exhaustive dynamic exercise. CIBA 82:42, 1981
45. Seliger V, Dolejs L, Karas V: Dynamometric comparison of maximum eccentric, concentric and isometric contractions using EMG and energy expenditure measurements. Eur J Appl Physiol 45:235, 1980
46. Rothstein JM: Measurement in Physical Therapy. Churchill Livingstone, New York, 1985
47. Ferreti A, Cerullo G, Russo G: Suprascapular neuropathy in volleyball. J Bone Joint Surg 69A:260, 1987
48. Bryan WJ, Wild JJ: Isolated infraspinatus atrophy. A common cause of posterior shoulder pain and weakness in throwing athletes. Am J Sports Med 17:130, 1989
49. Maitland GO: Vertebral Manipulation. 5th Ed. Butterworth (Publishers), London 1987

Appendix 5-1.
Research Abstracts

Albert MS: The biceps brachii long head tendon: biomechanics and a specific rehabilitation protocol. Submitted for publication, 1989.

Several important biomechanical roles of the long head of the biceps brachii tendon (LHBBT) in overhead sports activities indicate the need for specific high speed, eccentric biased rehabilitation. A functional clinical training program using inertial loading (Impulse) is described, with retrospective analysis of seventeen patient cases. The inertial protocol involves time phased resistance weight decreases to produce increased speed at the shoulder joint in a flexion pattern with slight elbow flexion maintained. Inertial training produced safe eccentric loads to the LHBBT with the capacity for forearm rotation and varied shoulder abduction positions and was an effective component of rehabilitation in this varied group of shoulder patients. Continued research of this protocol and the physiological effects of inertial training is warranted.

Malone TR: Inertial exercise system analysis through electro-myography, accelerometry and digital wave forms. 1989.

The Impulse (inertial exercise system) was developed through the work of Dr. William McLeod to allow acceleration and deceleration forces through the functional activity of overcoming resistance to movement (inertial forces). It consists of a trolley which moves along a reduced friction, track allowing reciprocal functional movement patterns. This was introduced to the physical therapy market in 1985 and allows the patient to experience rhythymic acceleration (overcoming the inertia) and deceleration (catching the moving trolley). Patients are able to use three protocols for this experience. The concept of this exercise is really of a neuro-muscular coordination pattern, and not a strengthening tool per se. Greater velocity results in greater force through the concept of mass × acceleration. Electromyographic analysis reveals an acceleration phase consisting of a concentric movement and an eccentric catch being present. The accelerometer demonstrates very high levels, particularly with lower weights and emphasizes the importance of neuromuscular efficiency. Clinical utilization of the device follows a pattern of developing control through teaching the exercise of the noninvolved extremity first. We typically use heavy weight with a sub-maximal activation level and allow a long travel of the trolley. After the patient becomes coordinated with this, one decreases the weight and increases the speed. We have seen excellent carryover to the opposite extremity and thus feel that the primary function of this device is in neuromuscular training.

6

Eccentric Isokinetics

PATRICIA A. HAGEMAN
TERESA A. SORENSEN

Advances in technology have led to the development of isokinetic muscle testing devices that allow eccentric exercise in addition to concentric activity. Despite the availability of these devices, research on appropriate isokinetic rehabilitation methods utilizing eccentric muscle training for various injuries or pathologies is limited and varied in nature.

An advantage of isokinetic exercise is that it provides a method of loading dynamically contracting muscles to capacity at a speed that may be manipulated. The muscle is able to maintain a state of maximum contraction through its full range, and so permit a maximal demand on its work capacity. Velocities may be set to allow the muscle to function relative to the dynamic conditions in some functional activity. The ability to offer eccentric isokinetic activity significantly contributes to the overall rehabilitation of an individual because eccentric muscular contractions play a major role in functional activities and athletics.[1,2]

The clinician, athletic trainer, and coach must be aware of the results of eccentric isokinetic research in order to safely apply eccentric isokinetic exercise in a preventative or rehabilitation program. Eccentric isokinetic activity differs from concentric isokinetic activity in the development of muscular force at various speeds. The force curves for concentric and eccentric contractions of the same muscle differ. Generally, the force generated during eccentric contractions exceeds the force developed during concentric activity at the same velocity and angle (Fig. 6-1). While this may lead to a conclusion that eccentric isokinetic training would be a most effective technique for maximal strength gains, the nature of eccentric muscular activity may place an individual at greater risk for muscular soreness or muscle damage.[3]

Other factors that must be considered when testing or training individuals using eccentric isokinetic activity include awareness of terminology and common methods for reporting objective data. Concerns for reliability of isokinetic measurements are important if the data collected are to be meaningful. Positions selected for testing and training will have a significant impact on torque production, and thus may traumatize a particular group of muscles. Proper orientation of the patient and other safety factors should be followed to prevent injuries. Caution is advised when making clinical decisions for functional activities based upon the results of data from eccentric isokinetic testing.

The purposes of this chapter are to discuss critical factors that affect eccentric isokinetic activities and to present guidelines for introducing eccentric isokinetic activities into rehabilitation and training programs.

ISOKINETICS

Definition

In theory, isokinetic devices test the ability of muscle groups to develop torque at a constant speed within and throughout a specified range of motion (ROM). Constant speed or isokinetic movements

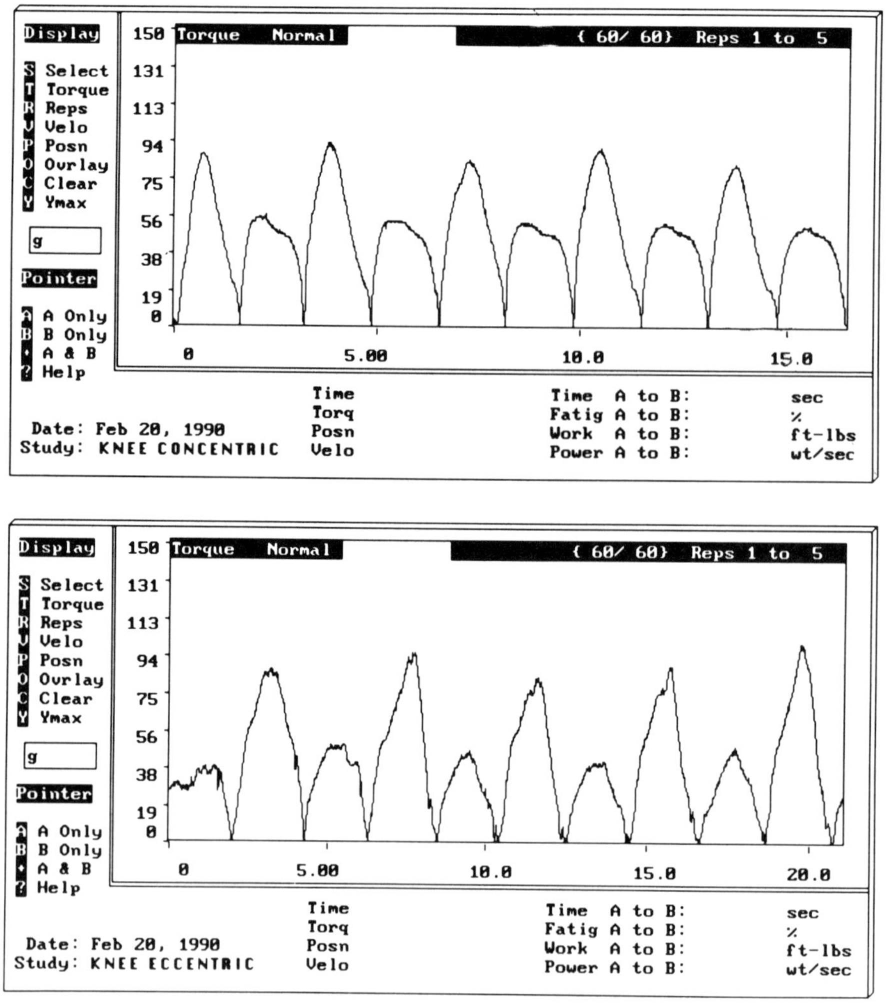

A

Fig. 6-1. **(A)** Concentric and eccentric torque curves of the quadriceps and hamstrings in a 20-year-old woman at a velocity of 60 degrees per second. (*Figure continues.*)

do not generally occur naturally; however, the advantage of constant speed testing is that a body segment is allowed to generate its maximum force or torque production throughout the ROM tested. Isokinetic devices allow activity at an average range of speeds from zero to 300 degrees per second and some offer velocities above 400 degrees per second. Many functional activities require movement faster than these ranges, up to ranges of 900 to 2,000 degrees per second depending upon the activity or sport.[4,5] Although the range of speeds available on isokinetic devices may not accommodate the fast velocities required of many activities, isokinetics allows some similarity to the type of muscular contractions needed in functional and athletic activities.

Isokinetic testing whether performed concentrically or eccentrically must be considered as another form of muscle testing. All forms of muscle testing including isokinetic testing appear to have limited use in predicting injury or functional capacity and the operator must be aware of this when making inferences to function or performance of the subjects tested.[6–8]

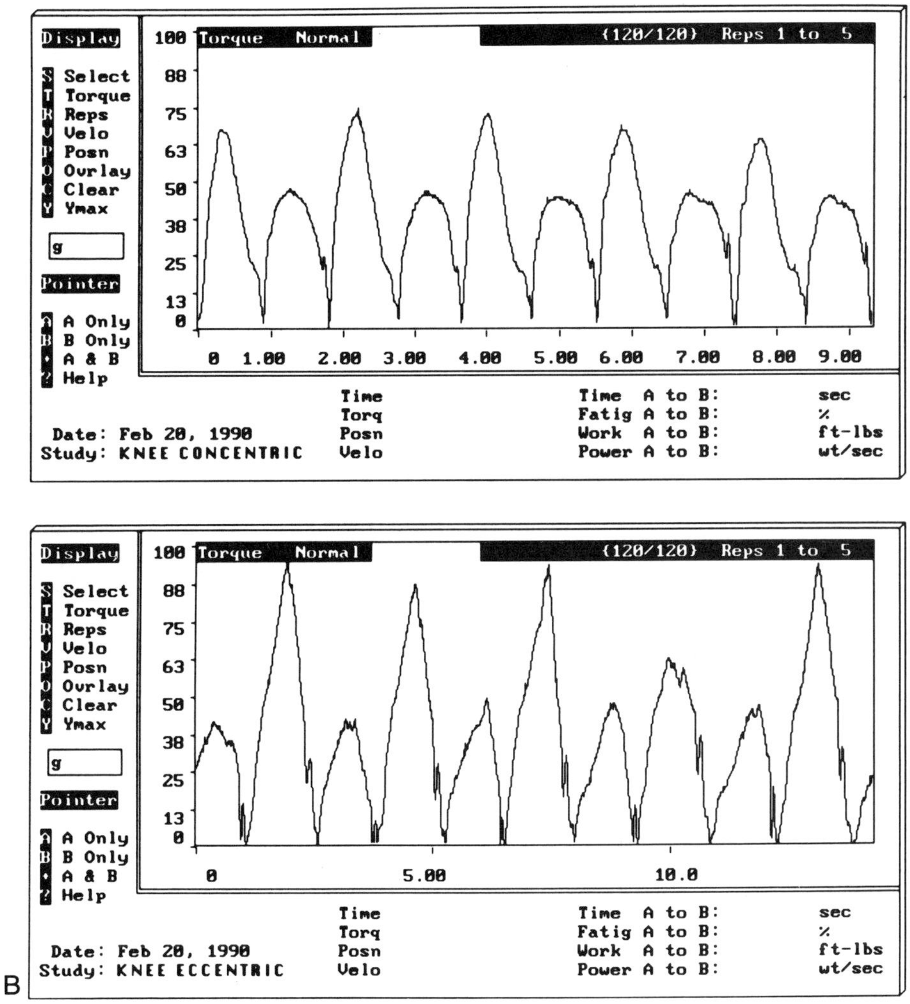

Fig. 6-1 (*Continued*). **(B)** Concentric and eccentric torque curves of the quadriceps and hamstrings in a 20-year-old woman at a velocity of 120 degrees per second.

Isokinetic Measurement

Rothstein et al.[9] critically analyzed the types of measurements and terms used for reporting isokinetic data and suggested that the proper terms reflecting isokinetic measurements are force, torque, work, and power. Torque is the force times the perpendicular distance from the axis for rotation (moment arm) to the line of application of that force, and is recorded in foot-pounds and/or newton-meters (1 foot-pound = 1.356 newton-meters; 1 newton-meter = .7375 foot-pounds). Absolute peak torque is the highest single value obtained during a series of repetitions and may be an appropriate indicator of an individual's maximum capability to generate torque. The mean value of a series of repetitions is also used as representative of an individual's maximum capacity.

Operational definitions of work and power are defined in several ways and comparison of reported value in the literature is difficult. Work is calculated as the area under the torque curve dur-

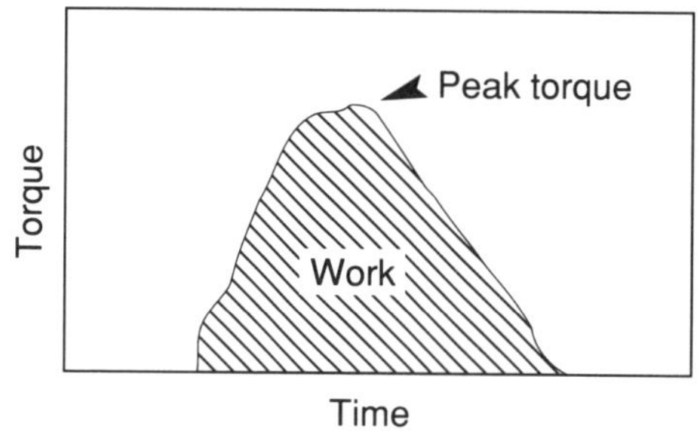

Fig. 6-2. Isokinetic peak torque and work. (From Morrissey,[61] with permission.)

ing a single isokinetic contraction or multiple contractions (Fig. 6-2). Power refers to the rate of doing work or the amount of work to be performed over time. Average power is the total work done by a force divided by the total time it takes the force to do the work. Power is recorded as watts.

Limb Comparison

Torque and/or force values of injured to uninjured limbs are reported as a ratio or percentage of deficit (Fig. 6-3). Clinicians often theorize that a torque discrepancy of 10 percent or more between the two extremities indicates the presence of a muscle imbalance that predisposes an extremity to injury. Conflicting results are found within the literature and this theory has not been substantiated.[10]

The majority of reasearch is based upon concentric isokinetic activity. No significant differences were found in torque values between knees in two separate studies that compared dominant and nondominant limbs of healthy adults during eccentric isokinetics exercise.[11,12] Specific comparisons of upper extremity muscle groups during eccentric isokinetic exercise are not available. Differences have been reported between torque values in dominant and nondominant upper extremities during concentric isokinetic activity.[13,14] Torque differences between upper extremities were attributed to training effects or repetitive use of the limb.

Although comparisons between extremities is a commonly accepted clinical practice, those who utilize both concentric and eccentric isokinetic testing must consider the principle of specificity of exercise and the nature of a functional activity. While comparisons of measurements between limbs may be the best guideline currently available for isokinetic evaluation, this practice may not be appropriate. Research has not clearly demonstrated that the muscle torque produced by both left and right extremities should be similar.

Ratios

Torque values obtained with isokinetic measurements often are expressed as ratios for agonist to antagonistic muscles or for comparisons of contraction types within the same muscle. The use of torque ratios for clinical judgements have caused concern. Many factors contribute to error in these ratios such as gravity or the methods used to calculate the ratios.

The most frequently reported ratio is the hamstrings to quadriceps torque ratio. Nosse[15] reviewed 50 reports pertaining to the concentrically produced hamstrings to quadriceps torque ratio and found that a wide range was considered normal (0.43 to 0.90) depending upon the population tested, velocity, isokinetic dynamometer, and testing populations used. A concensus for what is considered normal has not been established for any muscle group or for either concentric or eccentric isokinetic muscle contraction types.

One of the marketing points for using eccentric isokinetics is that the client who complains of musculoskeletal pain may have normal concentric function but altered eccentric function. Comparing concentric with eccentric torque is a widely accepted clinical practice. Bennett and Stauber[16] compared the eccentric to concentric torque pattern within a muscle group and described this as a ratio. They used this ratio to target subjects for an eccentric isokinetic training study. Subjects who demonstrated a 15 percent deficit of eccentric to concentric torque were selected to participate in eccentric training. Figure 6-4 illustrates the relative torque values in symptomatic and nonsymptomatic subjects. Trudelle-Jackson et al.[17] suggest that many asymptomatic individuals possess an eccentric to concentric deficit. Further study is

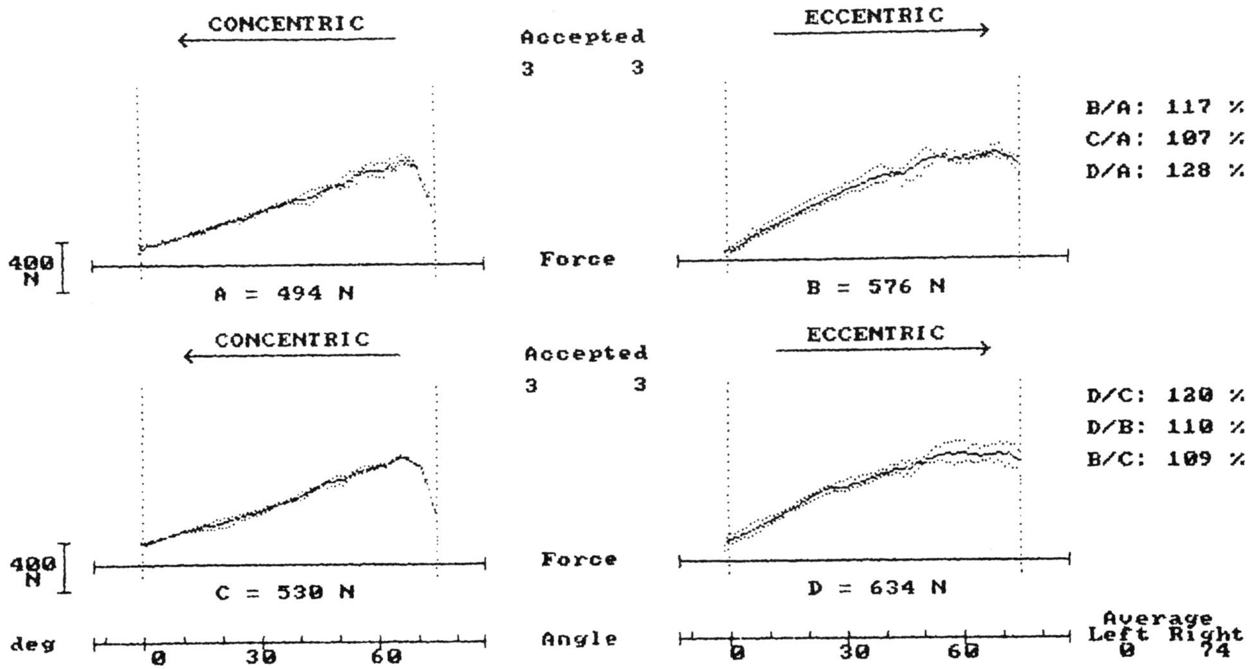

Fig. 6-3. Kin-Com average force ratios for the quadriceps in an 18-year-old man, 4 weeks following a medial collateral ligament sprain. *A*, concentric average force produced by the injured limb. *B*, eccentric average force produced by the injured limb. *C*, concentric average force produced by the uninjured limb. *D*, eccentric average force produced by the uninjured limb. The ratio D/B indicates that the injured limb tested 10 percent stronger than the uninjured limb during quadriceps testing eccentrically.

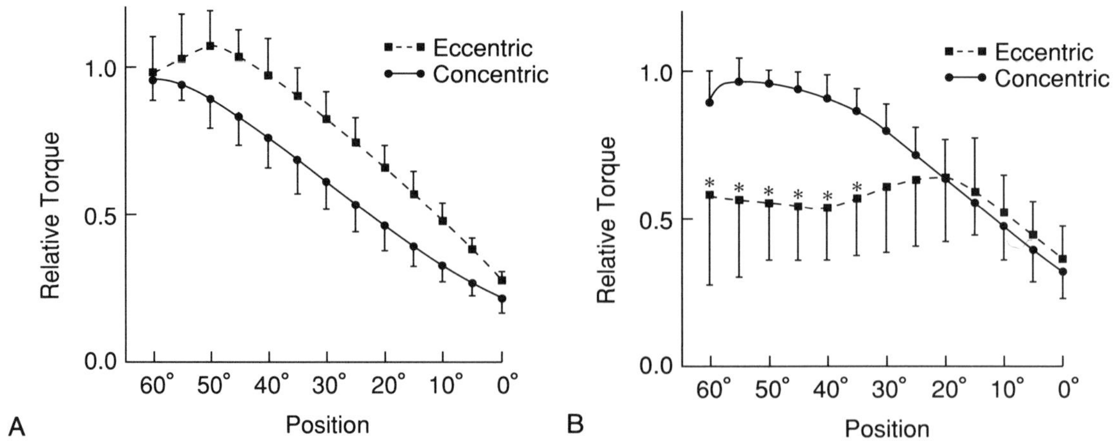

Fig. 6-4. Relative torque as a function of knee position for the extensor muscles during concentric and eccentric exercises. **(A)** The asymptomatic knee. **(B)** The symptomatic knee of patients with anterior knee pain syndrome. The data represent relative mean values ($N = 7$) ± 1 SD. (From Bennett and Stauber,[16] with permission.)

needed to identify the relationship between eccentric to concentric strength within a muscle group.

Reliability Issues

Because isokinetic devices offer a complete, concise printout of objective data, it may be easy for the operator to make a false assumption that the data obtained is reliable and accurately reflects the performance of the muscles. Test-retest reliability of isokinetic testing is crucial for obtaining meaningful data. Operators often incorrectly assume that the mechanical reliability of the device is the same as test-retest reliability. Several studies that examined the mechanical properties of the Cybex I (Cybex, Ronkonkoma, NY) and KIN-COM (Chattex Corp. Chattanooga, TN) have been used as references for the reliability and validity of isokinetic testing.[18–20] These studies tested a limited number of conditions and did not examine the reliability of test-retest measurements on either healthy subjects or relevant clinical populations. Validity of measurement cannot be demonstrated for a device but for the specific inferential use of the measurement.[21]

Factors that effect reliability include machine calibration, alignment of the joint axis to be tested, joint stabilization, positioning and testing protocols, therapist commands and methods, and subject cooperation and fatigue.

The axis of rotation of any body segment tested must be aligned with the axis of the machine used regardless of the type of device used or contraction types tested or else errors in isokinetic measurements will occur. The measurement error is less in joints where the axis of rotation moves only a small amount and limb segments may be stabilized easily, such as in testing the knee or elbow joints. Testing more complex joints such as the ankle, wrist, or shoulder may result in even larger errors because of the difficulty in stabilization and matching the true multiple axes of rotation occurring within the joints.

Devices such as the KIN-COM measure forces through the use of a force measurement transducer located at the point of force application. For these devices, distance measurements from the axis of rotation to the force pad must be made for torque calculations (Fig. 6-5). The operator of these devices must be aware that comparison of an individual's muscular force generation from a particular limb between time periods may differ if the force transducer is located at a different distance from the axis of rotation between testing periods.

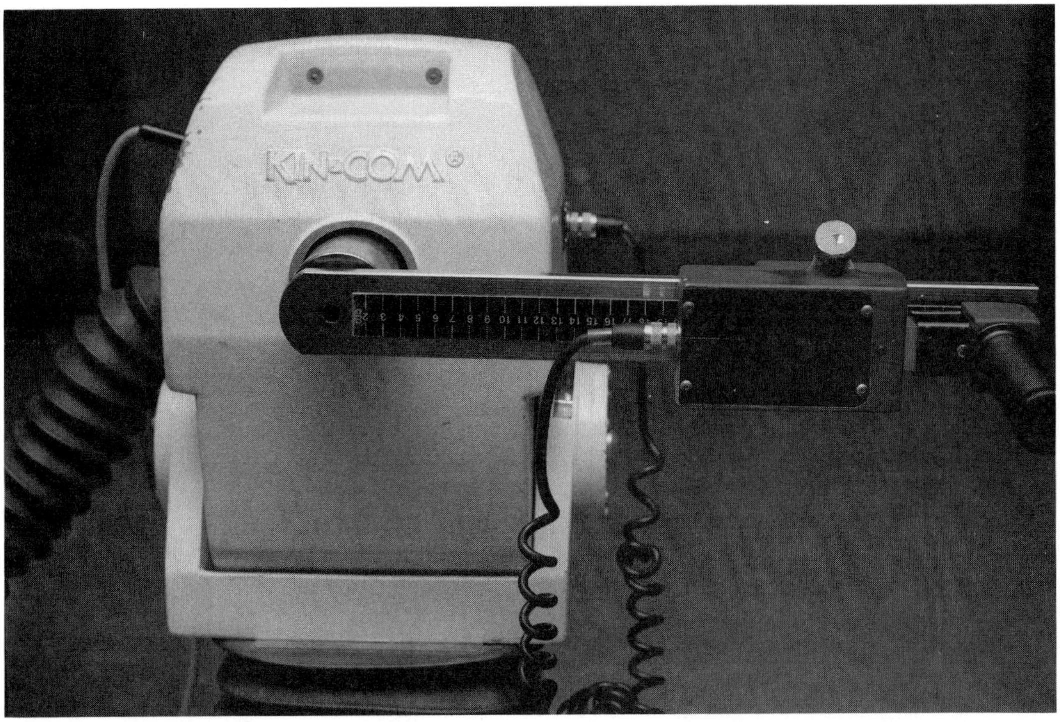

Fig. 6-5. Close-up of the force transducer and force pad on the Kin-Com. The length of the lever arm must be measured to calculate torque on the Kin-Com because the computer screen only displays force production.

Many devices calculate torque automatically through continuous monitoring of the force arm distance and the force produced. A study of quadriceps concentric torque production using the Cybex showed that force pad placement does effect the torque produced.[22] This has not been studied in devices offering eccentric isokinetic activity, however, clinicians should attempt to be consistent in positioning and force pad placement to improve test-retest reliability.

Several devices have attempted to accommodate the changing axis of rotation during testing by offering a sliding cuff attachment (Fig. 6-6). Whether this sliding cuff makes a difference in the torque values obtained is not clear based upon limited research.[23]

A wide range of test-retest reliability values are reported in the literature for both concentric and eccentric isokinetic measurements and these reliability values reflect a variety of procedures, protocols, and outcome criteria. Jackson et al.[24] examined the reliability of subjects performing two independent sets of three maximal concentric and eccentric contractions of the knee extensors at 50 degrees per second within the same day. Using the average torque of the three contractions as the outcome measure, they reported both concentric and eccentric measurements were reliable. High reliability for eccentric isokinetic contractions of the knee flexors was reported by Snow and Johnson[25] who tested at 30 and 180 degrees per second over 1 week.

Wessel et al.[26] studied the reliability of eccentric and concentric work measurements of the quadriceps at 60 and 180 degrees per second over two sessions, 1 week apart. The subjects performed six maximal eccentric contractions. No significant differences were found among trials or between weeks for the work measurement of concentric or eccentric contractions. Wessel et al.[26] reported

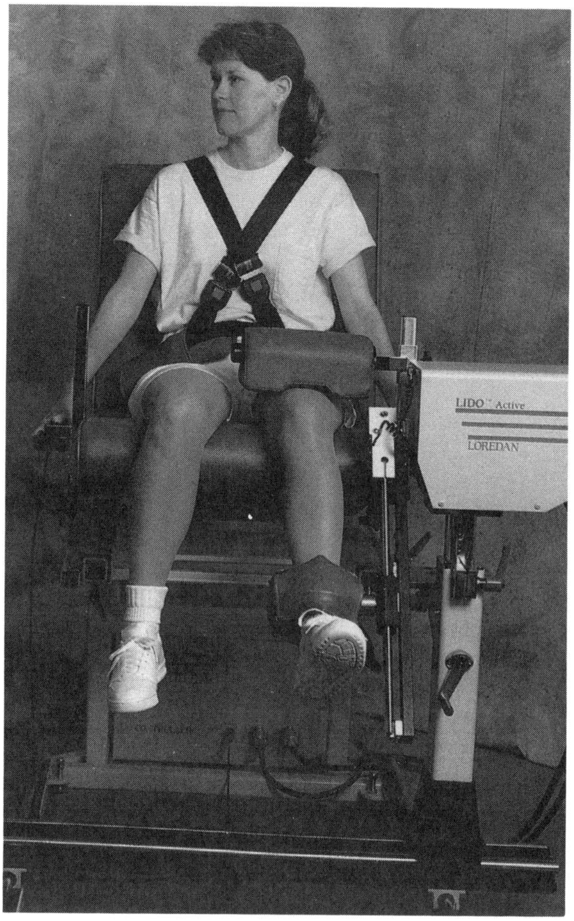

Fig. 6-6. The sliding cuff attachment on the Lido accommodates to the changing biologic lever arm during movement. (Courtesy of Loredan, Davis, CA.)

that the maximum of four to six trials was more reliable than any of the other measures when both contraction types at both velocities were considered.

The results of Wilhite et al.[27] suggest that testing order influences the degree of reliabilty at the higher speed of 180 degrees per second during concentric and eccentric isokinetic activity. They tested 18 subjects at three speeds of 60, 120, and 180 degrees per second in random fashion. Based upon the results they recommend that subjects be given longer practice periods performing high speeds and/or experience slower speeds prior to being tested at the high speeds.

Test-retest reliability for upper extremity eccentric isokinetic testing is low to fair based upon the results from studies of elbow flexors, and shoulder internal and external rotators in healthy adults.[28,29]

Based upon the research, test-retest reliability for the knee flexors and extensors appears to be high during concentric and eccentric isokinetic activity, but not for upper extremity exercise. Further research is needed to clearly establish the reliability of clinical testing for all joints. Operators of isokinetic devices should not assume that test-retest reliability is high for all methods used.

The effect of gravity on test results also produces distortion of the data.[30–32] Some devices attempt to correct for gravity through a computer software based algorithm. The operator must clarify whether subject data obtained were gravity corrected before making torque comparisons.

Comparison of Devices

The number of isokinetic dynamometer systems available has expanded rapidly. While most machines are designed to measure the same parameters, research has shown significant differences in values obtained from different machines.[33–35] Clinicians should not compare results from one isokinetic device with another. Normative data gathered from one device cannot be generalized for use with another testing system.

Force-Velocity Relationship

Eccentric produced torque is reported to increase as velocity increases, although conflicting results of the force-velocity relationship are found among eccentric isokinetic studies. Several researchers investigating elbow flexors reported muscular force increased as the velocity increased during eccentric activity.[28,36] The assumption that torque would increase significantly at higher speeds during eccentric activity was not clear according to Walmsley et al.[37] because they found a plateau effect when examining the mean peak torque of wrist extensors at specific joint angles.

A review of additional studies indicates that there is a trend toward increased force generation during eccentric isokinetics although this increase may not be significant. Hanten and Wieding[38] observed an increase in the force produced by the quadriceps from zero to 200 degrees per second during eccentric exercise, but this increase was not significant across the subsequent 11 velocities tested. Chandler and Duncan[39] investigated the quadriceps torque of 50 males at three velocities and found the eccentric force production remained nearly constant across the three velocities though the concentric force increased across the three velocities. Eloranta and Komi[40] found no clear difference in quadriceps eccentric force values between speeds, but the speeds tested were within a small range.

A study by Hageman et al.[11] also reported no significant differences in eccentric quadriceps or hamstrings torque between the speeds of 30 and 180 degrees per second (Fig. 6-7). The results of a study of shoulder internal and external rotators in two different positions were similar in that a significant increase in eccentric produced torque at the higher speed of 180 degrees per second was not found compared with 60 degrees per second.[29]

The research implies that clinicians may expect the torque to increase as the velocity increases, however, this increase may not be significant. Examples of eccentric isokinetic force-velocity patterns of the quadriceps are illustrated in Figure 6-8. Current practice involves involves testing at the lower speeds and gradual progression to faster speeds. Until research more clearly defines the force-velocity relationship, caution is advised when introducing the subjects to higher speeds. Factors such as orientation to eccentric activity, gradual progression of eccentric programs, and the time following an injury prior to initiating ec-

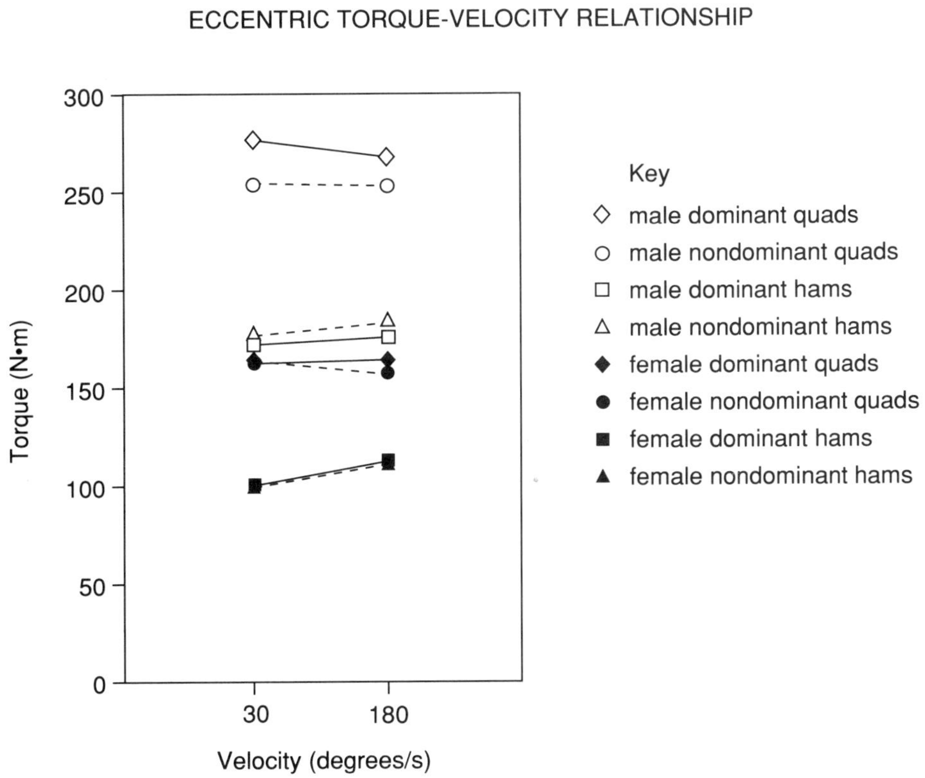

Fig. 6-7. Torque-velocity relationship from the quadriceps during eccentric contractions for males ($n = 12$) and for females ($n = 13$) at two test speeds. (From Hageman et al.,[11] with permission.)

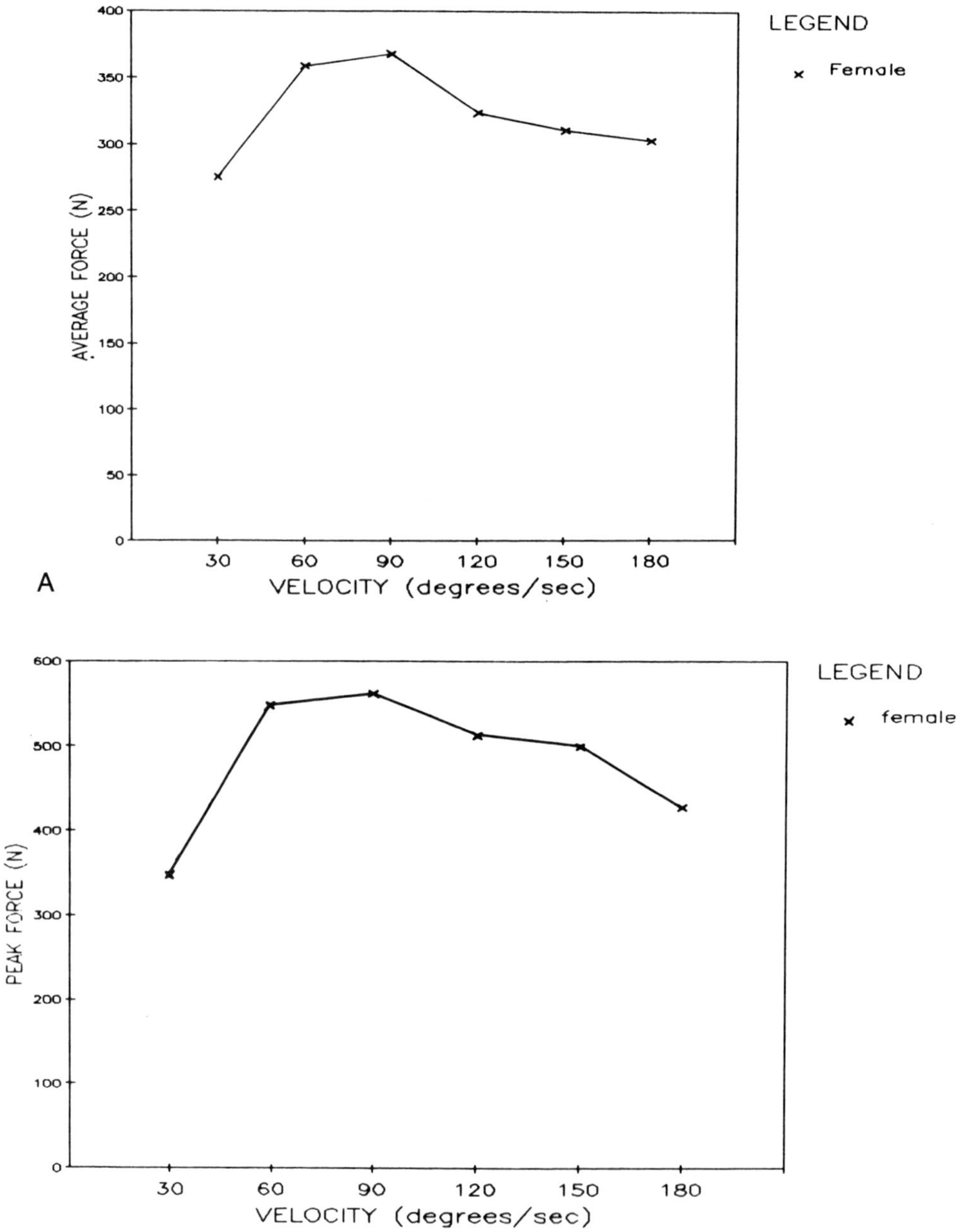

Fig. 6-8. **(A)** Average and **(B)** peak force-velocity relationships from the quadriceps during eccentric and concentric exercise in a healthy 21-year-old woman.

centric isokinetics may be more crucial when introducing the subject to higher speeds than the actual use of higher speeds.

Positioning

Positioning may be a key factor in development of torque values for any given joint. This concept has been supported during both concentric and eccentric isokinetic activities.[29,41–45] Factors explaining these differences found in torque production among various positions are attributed to the change in the length/tension ratios of the musculature involved and gravitational forces affecting the joints tested.

The operator of isokinetic devices should consider the arthrokinematics of the joint involved and the actual pathology of a patient prior to selection of an isokinetic training position for safety and optimal training. For example, if the patient has recurrent anterior dislocation of the shoulder, the positioning for initial eccentric training that places the shoulder at high risk for dislocation should be avoided.

Training during eccentric isokinetic training would in theory be optimal if the positioning was similar to the functional activity targeted for improvement. Further research is needed to identify optimal isokinetic training positions.

Overflow Training

An overflow phenomenon was observed in a study by Ellenbecker et al.[1] who examined the results of a 6 week isokinetic training program of the shoulder internal and external rotators in 22 varsity tennis players. The players were divided into two training groups either eccentric training or concentric training. Training consisted of 6 sets of 10 repetitions using the velocity spectrum pyramidal order concept (60, 180, 210, 180, 60 degrees per second). The group that trained eccentrically resulted in significant concentric strength gains, and eccentric isokinetic training produced greater increases in concentric strength than concentric isokinetic training. The eccentrically trained group did not demonstrate significant gains in eccentric isokinetic strength except during external rotation at 210 degrees per second. This result was attributed to the induced soreness during the 6 week training period that might have prohibited maximal tension gain.

The concern for risk of injury during eccentric exercise and the production of delayed onset muscle soreness (DOMS) led Hay and Feuerbach[46] to compare the effects of concentric training on the peak torques exerted by the elbow flexors acting concentrically and eccentrically. Thirty-five subjects participated in concentric training of the elbow flexors at 60 degrees per second over 6 weeks. Their findings indicated that concentric training was equally effective in increasing concentric and eccentric peak torques; however, a control group was not used and concentric and eccentric training occurred at different speeds of 60 and 40 degrees per second, respectively.

Overflow training was not reported by Nicely et al.[47] who compared the effects of three types of isokinetic quadriceps training in a group of 27 females over 6 weeks. They reported that each training group (isokinetic-concentric, isokinetic-eccentric, or isometric) scored significantly higher only in the type of contraction in which they trained supporting the theory of specificity.

Subjects who participated in a 7 week eccentric isokinetic training program at 60 degrees per second increased their values of peak torque at both 60 degrees per second and at 180 degrees per second.[48] The implications of this study were that training eccentrically at one speed may result in improvements of torque values at other speeds.

Additional study seems necessary to clearly define overflow training between concentric and eccentric exercise. Further investigations also need to focus on developing training guidelines for using eccentric isokinetics. The results of clinical observation show that patients benefit from using a combination of both eccentric and concentric isokinetic exercise. The rationale for using a combination of eccentric and concentric isokinetic exercise is that most functional and sports activities involve concentric and eccentric muscular contractions.

Fatigue During Eccentric Activity

Research results are not clear about whether a muscle fatigues more rapidly during eccentric or concentric contractions. Komi et al.[49–50] found that a muscle fatigues at a much greater extent when exercised eccentrically at low velocities than it does when exercised concentrically. Gray and Chandler[51] reported a 0.3 percent decline in quadriceps peak torque production during 20 repetitions of eccentric exercise compared with a 47.7 percent decrease during concentric exercise. Significant fatigue was reported by DeNuccio et al.[52] using a protocol of 40 repetitions during both eccentric (30.3 percent decline) and concentric (13.7 percent decline) testing of the quadriceps.

These studies differed in their methods and results, raising additional questions about the fatiguability of muscle during eccentric and concentric exercise. Komi et al.[49,50] tested forearm flexors, quadriceps, and glutei using lower velocities whereas Gray and Chandler[51] and DeNuccio et al.[52] tested the quadriceps at 180 degrees per second. Further testing is needed to define muscle fatigue during eccentric isokinetic activity.

Safety Concerns

Prior to implementing isokinetic eccentric exercise as a mode of testing or training, the operator must consider this form of exercise as an *adjunct* to a rehabilitation program. Safety factors to consider when using eccentric isokinetics include (1) timing of eccentric isokinetic introduction and use, (2) orientation of the subject to eccentric isokinetics, (3) preload and torque limit settings, (4) velocity, (5) joint position and ROM, (6) number of sets and repetitions, (7) physician recommendations, (8) manufacturer recommendations, and (9) machine shutdown.

Time

Because of the higher risk of muscle soreness and trauma during eccentric isokinetics, waiting until an injury has progressed to a nonacute phase is recommended. Eccentric isokinetics can exacerbate the exisiting injury or create new damage if given too soon or too forcibly. Eccentric activity involves greater tension per muscle fiber and may cause mechanical damage to the muscle, which is more extensive 30 hours postexercise. Walsmley et al.[37] suggest that eccentric contractions within 30 hours of an injury would exacerbate any trauma already present. Most clinical applications introduce eccentric isokinetics in the nonacute phase and after concentric isokinetics is tolerated. Eccentric isokinetics should be initiated with low intensity, fewer repetitions, and lower speeds (30 degrees per second).

Orientation of the Subject

Eccentric isokinetic movements may feel unnatural to the subject. The concept that a machine can push a limb when an individual pushes into the force pad may seem strange or awkward, and extra orientation may be necessary for introducing eccentric isokinetics to any individual, especially one with an injury. Adequate warmup should be completed prior to eccentric isokinetic exercise. Recommendations for starting any testing procedure would include instructing the subject to contract isometrically against the resistance pad during a passive mode setting at 10 to 30 degrees per second; beginning actual eccentric isokinetics at a slow velocity of 30 to 60 degrees per second before advancing to a faster velocity; and testing the unaffected limb, which provides the subject with feedback as to the nature of eccentric isokinetics prior to testing an affected extremity.

Preload and Torque Limit Setting

The subject tested must provide an effort for the machine to operate during both concentric and eccentric isokinetic activity. If the subject voluntarily stops, the machine will also stop. Designs for isokinetic devices that permit eccentric activity include a robotic component that responds to subject impact. A concern for eccentric testing is that the machine must be set for a high enough threshold so that merely resting a body part on the machine will not trigger the device to move against the subject, especially if the subject is not prepared. The preload threshold is extremely important at higher speeds because the subject tested may be surprised at the quickness of movement and respond automatically generating high forces which may overstrain the muscles.

For safety reasons always adjust the device for a preload so that an effort must be made by the subject to trigger movement in the machine. The threshold force may vary between joints and individuals. Common threshold forces used are 20 to 50 newtons for upper extremity and 50 to 100 newtons for lower extremity.

Most devices feature a torque limit, which is established to stop the machine if the subject exceeds the preset torque limit. Differences exist between devices for upper torque limits. For example, the Kin-Com will automatically shutdown if a force of 2,000 newtons of force is exerted, although the operator may selectively adjust the shutdown force to a lower value. The Biodex (Biodex Corp, Shirley, NY) has an operator control to restrict torque development at a range of up to 150 foot-pounds of torque, or up to 300 ft-lb in some models. The LIDO (Loredan, Davis, CA) allows the operator to set a maximum eccentric load that is constantly responsive and appropriate to the patient's varying levels of performance. The maximum eccentric load is established by using feedback from the concentric effort produced by the patient.

These features, although different between devices, are designed to prevent the subject or patient from developing extremely high torque and to encourage submaximal effort by the patient.

Velocity

During most rehabilitation programs, eccentric isokinetics should be initiated at the slower velocities (30 to 60 degrees per second) before progressing to faster velocities. Athletes generally tolerate eccentric testing and training at higher velocities than the general population. Current eccentric training programs used clinically involve velocities up to 120 degrees per second for upper and lower extremity activities in the general population and up to 180 degrees per second in the athletic population.

Joint Positioning/Range of Motion

Clinical judgement should be used when positioning a subject, especially if the subject is rehabilitating from an injury. Studies have shown that position may significantly alter the amount of torque produced at any particular joint.[29,41–45] The joint kinematics should be normal before initiating any eccentric isokinetic exercise. Palpation of the joint is recommended during the eccentric isokinetic activity to confirm normal tracking of movement within the joint. Eccentric isokinetic training within a painfree ROM is recommended and the majority of machines allow restriction of movement. Certain joint motions usch as shoulder flexion and shoulder abduction tend to be uncomfortable because of the tendency for the axis of rotation of the shoulder to shift from the axis of rotation of the machine. By keeping the shoulder ROM restricted (less than 90 degrees) the axes of rotation are matched and the patient tolerates the activity.

Number of Sets and Repetitions

Warmup activities should be completed prior to any eccentric isokinetic exercise. Many devices are capable of a variety of programs such as concentric/eccentric reciprocal training patterns or eccentric/eccentric patterns. Sorensen (unpublished clinical data, 1986-1990) recommends that the concentric/eccentric pattern be used because subjects adapt to the pattern more readily than others.

A limited number of repetitions is appropriate during eccentric isokinetic exercise because it is used as an adjunct form of exercise in a rehabilitation program. An average number of 30 repetitions is used for one muscle group, although some muscle groups adapt to training up to 90 repetitions (hamstrings). Initially, some patients only tolerate 10 to 30 repetitions. Eccentric isokinetic workouts are clinically viewed as optimal at three times per week preferably with a day rest between sessions. Rest periods between contractions should be patient and symptom guided. The use of ice or cold packs after the eccentric isokinetic rehabilitation program may reduce and/or prevent muscle inflammation or soreness.

Consulting With the Physician

Consulting with the physician prior to initiating eccentric isokinetic rehabilitation is advised, especially for all patients who had surgery. The clinician should be aware of the nature and extent of all surgeries when determining the intensity of the eccentric isokinetic training.

Manufacturer's Recommendations

Manufacturer's recommendations for setup, stabilization, and use of any device should be followed to ensure safety during operation. All personnel using the robotic dynamometers must be fully trained to prevent injuries when operating the devices.

Machine Shutdown

It has been our experience that if the Kin-Com machine detects a velocity, angle, or force error during training or testing, the power will automatically turn off and the arm will lock up. The arm will not move until the Kin-Com is turned on from the main menu screen. This process takes a few seconds. This type of shutdown problem, which results in an abrupt stop of the patient limb, has made the authors cautious about training or testing at speeds higher than 200 to 300 degrees per second. This shutdown has not been a problem at lower speeds.

Precautions and Contraindications

Debilitated patients and/or patients with total joint replacements are not candidates for eccentric isokinetic testing. Patients with neuromuscular diseases that cause poor motor control are also poor candidates for eccentric isokinetic testing. Soft tissue healing constraints, acute strains, severe pain, marked effusion, unstable joints, or unstable fractures are considered absolute contraindications for eccentric isokinetic activity.

In all uses, the operator of the isokinetic device must use sound clinical judgement prior to using eccentric isokinetic exercise with patients or clients.

CLINICAL APPLICATIONS

The remaining portion of this chapter discusses clinical applications for isokinetic training. These applications are *not* all inclusive but are intended to serve as guidelines or as a point of reference for clinicians, trainers, and coaches who are beginning to incorporate eccentric isokinetic activity as part of a rehabilitation program. Persons using these applications must use their individual judgements when deciding to use these ideas or protocols in any particular situation.

KNEE JOINT

The majority of articles and protocols found on eccentric isokinetic activity are focused on the knee joint perhaps because the knee is a commonly injured joint. Current examples for eccentric isokinetic programs for nonsurgical and surgical knee diagnoses are included in Tables 6-1 and 6-2. Common positions used for knee testing are seated or prone (Fig. 6-9).

Nonsurgical Diagnoses

Anterior Knee Pain

Bennett and Stauber[16] found that within 130 patients with various knee disorders that produced symptoms of anterior knee pain, 41 patients demonstrated a suppression in torque production during eccentric exercise and generally in the portion of the ROM between 30 and 60 degrees of knee flexion ($P < .05$). The 41 patients participated in a training program three times per week involving concentric/eccentric exercises of the knee extensors at various speeds (30, 60, and 90 degrees per second) with the majority demonstrating relief of pain and torque deficiency after 2 to 4 weeks of training.

The rehabilitation program used by Bennett and Stauber[16] consisted of using a painfree ROM that was adjusted with each training session but was initially less than 50 degrees of knee flexion. Three sets of 10 repetitions at each of the following constant velocity settings (30, 60, and 90 degrees per second) were performed for a total of 90 repeti-

Table 6-1. Eccentric Isokinetic Programs for Nonsurgical Knee Diagnoses

Diagnosis or Symptom	Muscle Group	Program Progression	Special Precautions
Bennett and Stauber[16]			
Anterior knee pain	Knee extensors	3 sets of 10 reps Velocity (30°, 60°, 90°/s)	90 reps max per session Painfree ROM Initially <50° knee flexion
Jenson and DiFabio[53]			
Patellar tendonitis	Knee extensors	Initially 6 sets of 5 reps at 30°/s; weeks 2–8, 4 sets of 5 reps at each velocity Week 2: 30°, 35°/s Week 3: 30°, 35°, 40°/s Week 4: 30°, 40°, 45°/s Week 5: 30°, 40°, 50°/s Week 6: 30°, 45°, 60°/s Week 7: 30°, 50°, 65°/s Week 8: 30°, 50°, 70°/s	
Sorensen (unpublished clinical data, 1986-1990)			
Patellar tendonitis Chondromalacia Patellar malalignment	Knee extensors	Initially 3 sets of 10 reps at 30°/s Gradual progression to 3 sets of 10 reps at each speed (30°, 60°, 90°/s) Athletes may tolerate 120°/s	Patellar tracking must be stable Painfree ROM 90 reps maximum per session
Patellar subluxation	Knee extensors	General progression to 3 sets of 10 reps at 30°/s	Patellar tracking must be stable
Medial and lateral collateral ligament sprains	Knee extensors	Initially 3 sets of 10 reps at 30°/s Gradual progression to 3 sets of 10 reps at each speed (30°, 60°, 90°/s) Athletes may tolerate 120°/s	Begin after 2–6 weeks postinjury when pain, ROM, and effusion permit 90 reps maximum per session for the quadriceps
	Knee flexors	Initially 3 sets of 10 reps at 30°/s Gradual progression to 3 sets of 10 reps at each speed (30°, 60°, 90°, 120°/s) Athletes may tolerate 180°/s	
ACL sprain	Knee flexors	Initially 3 sets of 10 reps at 30°/s; progress to 3 sets of 10 reps at each velocity (30°, 60°, 90°, 120°/s) Athletes may tolerate 180°/s	Begin after 2–6 weeks postinjury when pain, ROM, and effusion permit Limit terminal extension

Abbreviations: ACL, anterior crucial ligament; ROM, range of motion.

tions per session. They allowed their patients to establish the rest intervals. The threshold force was a minimum of 50 newtons and was increased throughout the training period to ensure compliance.

Patellar Tendonitis

Jensen and DiFabio reported that eccentric exercise was an effective treatment for patients with patellar tendonitis.[53] In the subjects who participated in an 8 week eccentric isokinetic program (Table 6-1), the quadriceps femoris muscle work capacity increased. They commented that knee pain may limit the gains in strength.

Sorensen Protocols

Since June 1986, Sorensen (unpublished clinical data, 1986–1990) has developed and implemented an eccentric isokinetic exercise using the Kin-Com for rehabilitation programs in over 1,000

Table 6-2. Sorensen Eccentric Isokinetic Programs for Surgical Knee Diagnoses

Surgery	Muscle Group	Program Progression	Special Precautions
Lateral release	Knee extensors	Begin when pain and effusion permit, usually 4–6 weeks postop Initially use passive mode at 10°/s Progress to 3 sets of 10 reps at 30°/s Gradual progression to 3 sets of 10 reps at each speed (30°, 60°, 90°/s) Athletes may tolerate 120°/s	Avoid the painful range
Repair for patellar subluxation	Knee extensors	Very individualized Slow progression; similar to program for lateral release Maximum speeds recommended are 90°/s for general population 120°/s for athlete population	Follow physician orders Time reference to begin depends on extent of surgery
Arthroscopic surgery for removal of cartilage and scar tissue	Knee extensors Knee flexors	Similar to lateral release Begin when pain and effusion permit usually 2–6 weeks postop Begin with 3 sets of 10 reps at 30°/s Gradual progression to 3 sets of 10 reps at each speed (30°, 60°, 90°, 120°/s) up to 180°/s in athletes	
Patellectomy	Knee extensors	Begin when pain and effusion permit Begin in passive mode at 10°/s Progress to isokinetics at 30°/s up to 60°/s and on rare occasions up to 90°/s	Some patients may not tolerate isokinetic eccentric loading of quadriceps
ACL reconstruction (with or without cartilage repair)	Knee flexors	Usually introduced 4 weeks postop Initially 3 sets of 10 reps at 30°/s; progress to 3 sets of 10 reps at each velocity (30°, 60°, 90°, 120°/s) Athletes may tolerate 180°/s	Consult with physician Limit terminal extension

Abbreviations: ACL, anterior cruciate ligament.

patients, the majority being knee rehabilitation. The following programs for various diagnoses have been implemented with a clinical record of significant patient improvement and injuryfree training.

Patellofemoral Dysfunction

Patients with patellofemoral dysfunction, patellar tendonitis, malalignment of the patella, and chondromalacia may benefit from the addition of eccentric isokinetic training to the established rehabilitation program when they can perform concentric isokinetic exercise without pain. If the patient has difficulty with muscle control, introduce eccentrics using the passive mode at 10 degrees per second. Instruct the patient to push against the pad and submaximally resist its movement. Once the patient appears to understand the movement, eccentric isokinetics may be started at 30 degrees per second using approximately 3 sets of 10 repetitions or patient symptom guidance. Generally, most patients progress rapidly to a program involving 3 sets of 10 repetitions at 30, 60, and 90 degrees per second. Athletes could progress to 120 degrees per second of eccentric isokinetic loading of the quadriceps with precaution.

Patellar Subluxation

Patellar subluxation (nonsurgical) follows the above protocol with additional precautions. Eccentric isokinetic exercise should always be ac-

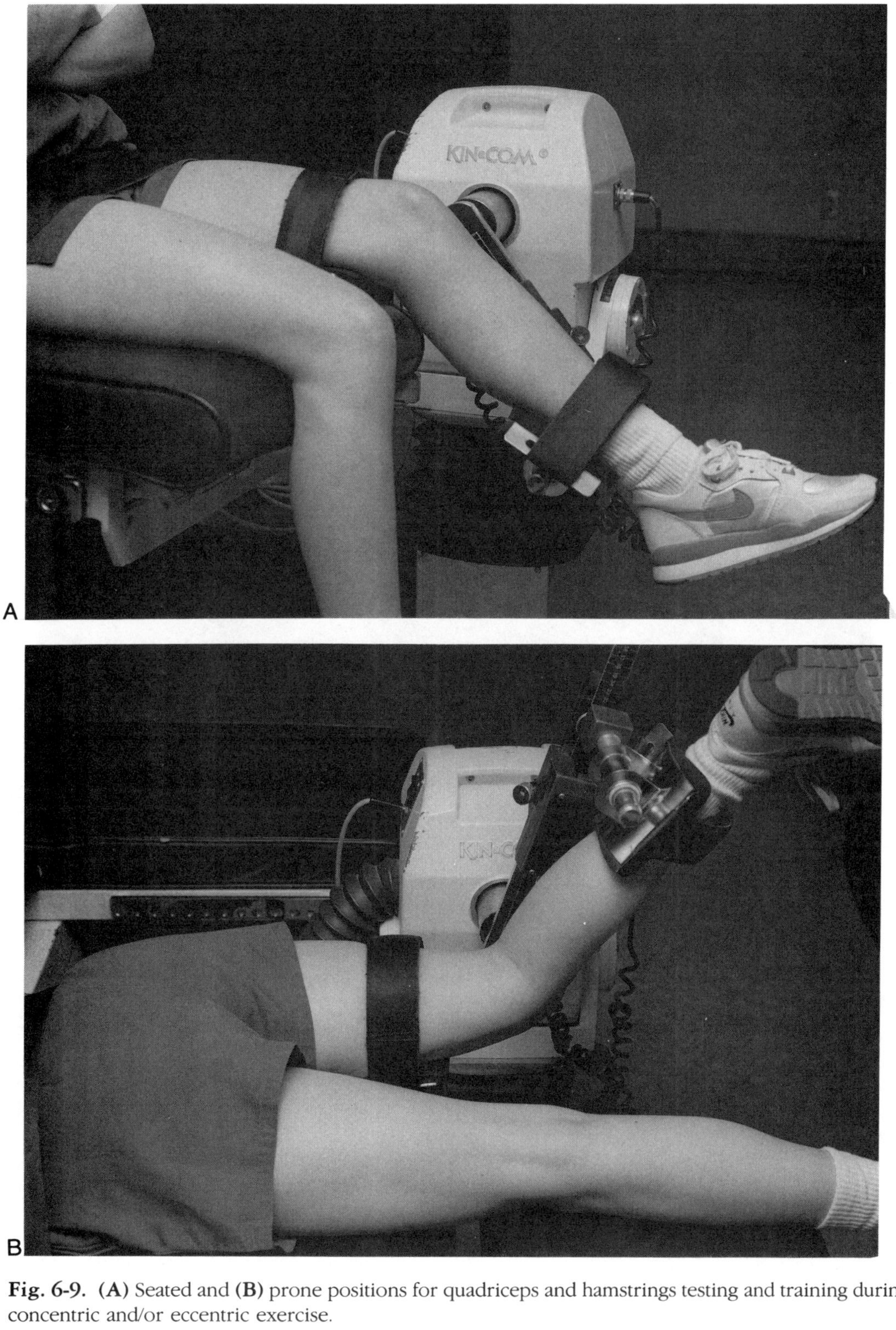

Fig. 6-9. **(A)** Seated and **(B)** prone positions for quadriceps and hamstrings testing and training during concentric and/or eccentric exercise.

companied by manual palpation over the patella to feel for subluxation (Fig. 6-10). The patella tracking should be stable before introducing this exercise. Eccentric isokinetic exercises are generally introduced at 4 to 6 weeks postdislocation. Patients frequently can only tolerate 3 sets of 10 repetitions at 30 degrees per second.

Medial or Lateral Collateral Tears

Use of adjustable knee braces allow for early eccentric isokinetic rehabilitation compared with the more conservative treatment technique of casting. Eccentric isokinetics of the quadriceps or hamstrings may be initiated for medial or lateral collateral tears (nonsurgical) between 2 to 6 weeks postinjury if the knee is braced depending on the patient's pain tolerance, active ROM of the knee, effusion, and physician approval. Sorensen protocol introduces the patient to eccentric isokinetic activity at 30 degrees per second working up to maximum velocities of 90 and 120 degrees per second for the quadriceps of nonathletes and athletes, respectively. Rehabilitation of the hamstrings usually is built up to 3 sets of 10 repetitions at 30, 60, 90, and 120 degrees per second in nonathletes and up to 180 degrees per second for athletes.

Anterior Cruciate Ligament Sprains

Patients with anterior cruciate ligament (ACL) strains (nonsurgical) also may also begin eccentric isokinetic training of the hamstrings when effusion and pain permit within 2 to 6 weeks postinjury. If significant knee joint instability is present, do not train the quadriceps using eccentric isokinetics. Introduce all exercise at 30 degrees per second. Terminal extension should be restricted so the patients train in the range of 30 to 90 degees knee motion. The sets, repetitions, and velocities used for hamstring training involves working up

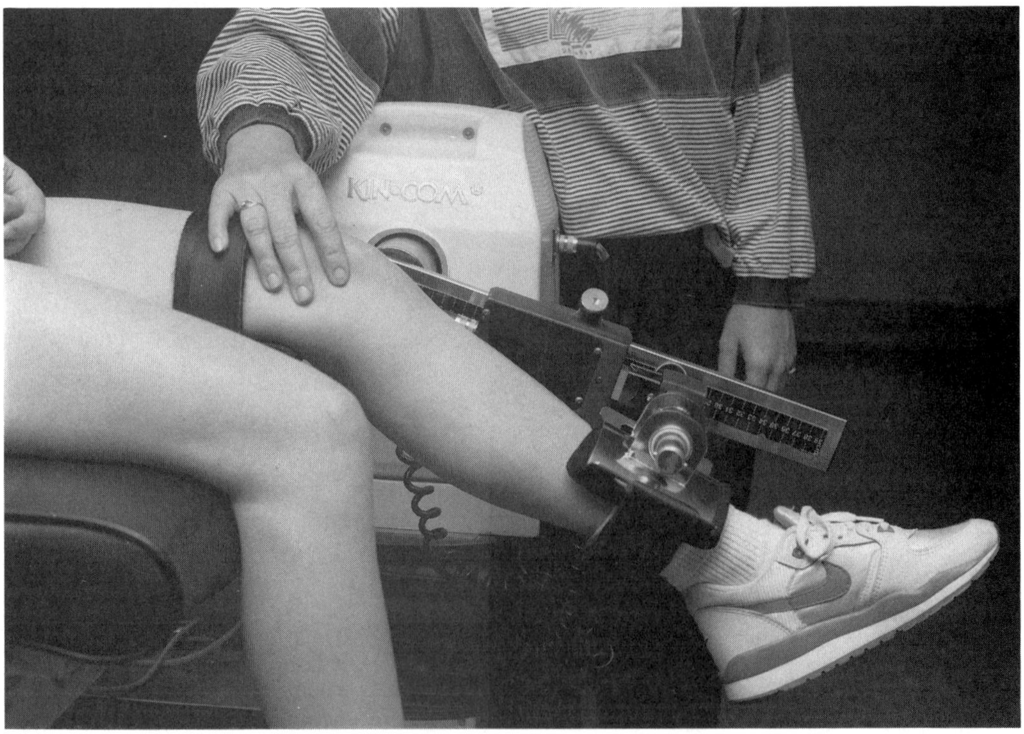

Fig. 6-10. Therapist palpating the patella prior to and during eccentric isokinetic activity to confirm patellar stability.

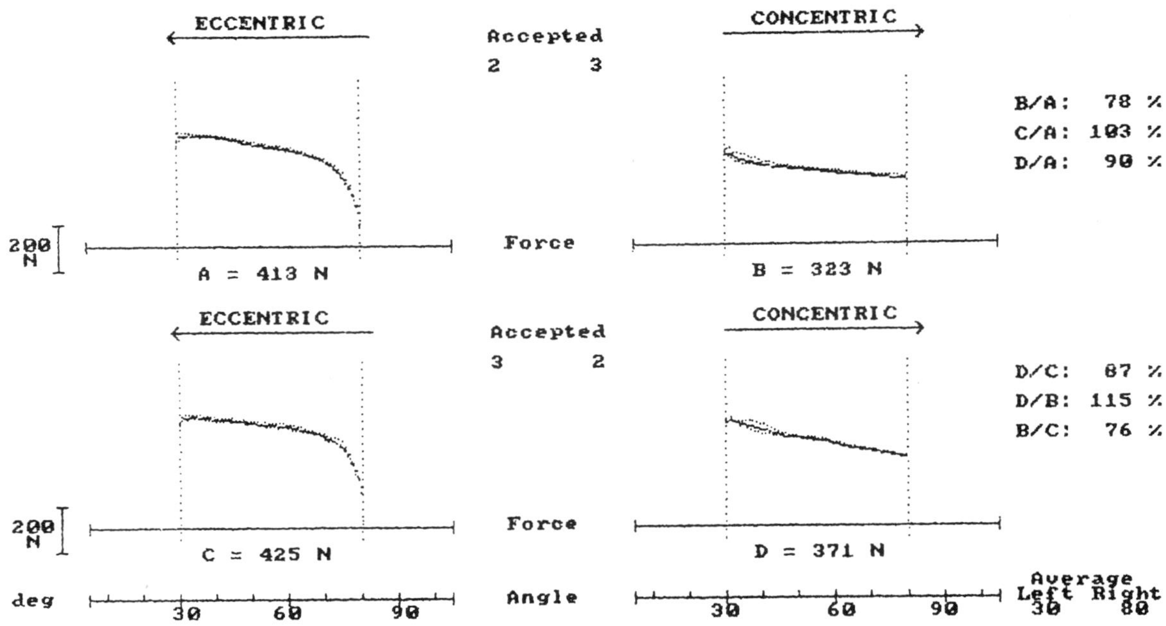

Remarks : RIGHT HAMSTRING TESTED 03% STRONGER THAN LEFT ECCENTRICALLY
RIGHT HAMSTRING TESTED 15% STRONGER THAN LEFT CONCENTRICALLY

Fig. 6-11. Kin-Com force curves for the hamstrings tested at 30 degrees per s in an 18-year-old woman 12 weeks following anterior cruciate ligament repair. *A*, eccentric average force produced by the injured limb; *B*, concentric average force produced by the injured limb; *C*, eccentric average force of the uninjured limb; *D*, concentric average force of the uninjured limb. Note that terminal extension was restricted.

to 3 sets of 10 repetitions at 30, 60, 90, and 120 degrees per second in nonathletes and up to 180 degrees per second in athletes.

Postsurgical Knees

The clinician should consult with the physician prior to introducing eccentric isokinetics into a patient's rehabilitation program following any surgery. Most eccentric isokinetic exercise may be initiated if the patient tolerates concentric isokinetic activity. The time reference for beginning eccentric isokinetics depends upon the extent of the surgery, the effusion present, the ROM, and the patient's pain tolerance.

The orientation and velocity suggestions for using eccentric isokinetics are similar for most surgeries. Introduce eccentric training of the quadriceps by using the passive mode at 10 degrees per second. The maximum speeds tolerated by the quadriceps generally are 90 degrees per second for the nonathlete, and 120 degrees per second for the athlete. Most rehabilitation begins at 30 degrees per second. Table 6-2 summarizes suggested protocols for surgical knees.

Repair for Patellar Subluxation

The protocols for using eccentric isokinetics should be very individualized for the patient following surgical repair for patellar subluxation and the clinician should coordinate planning of the rehabilitation program with the physician. Special attention should be directed at the tracking of the patella.

Arthroscopic Surgery and Lateral Release

Begin eccentric isokinetic training of the quadriceps when pain and effusion permit usually 4 to 6 weeks postoperatively.

Patellectomy

Eccentric isokinetic training may not be tolerated by all patients who have had a patellectomy. Training may be performed at 30 and 60 degrees per second but rarely is tolerated at 90 degrees per second.

Anterior Cruciate Ligament Repair

Sorensen adds eccentric isokinetic training of the hamstrings to the established rehabilitation program approximately 4 weeks postoperatively following ACL repair. The physician must be consulted prior to introducing the eccentric isokinetic training as physician concepts and surgical procedures may vary. Introduce the program for hamstrings at 30 degrees per second and then progress up to 3 sets of 10 repetitions at each speed of 30, 60, 90, and 120 degrees per second. Athletes may tolerate up to 180 degrees per second. An example of a patient test results 12 weeks postoperatively is displayed in Figure 6-11.

Indelicato and Huegel[54] published a protocol for using eccentric isokinetic training following a postsurgical repair of the ACL. They recommend beginning eccentric isokinetic work of the hamstrings at 6 weeks postoperatively. Indelicato and Huegel's recommendations are based upon use of the Biodex. They instruct the patient to resist the machine moving to extension from flexion in the passive mode at 60 degrees per second, because this prevents the system from shutting down when more than 150 foot-pounds of torque is exerted.

SHOULDER

The majority of research on eccentric isokinetic exercise for the shoulder is based upon the rotator mucle groups. The use of eccentric isokinetics for training the shoulder flexors or abductors is appropriate; however, eccentric isokinetic training may prove uncomfortable and awkward for the patient when attempting these exercises over a large ROM. This discomfort may be attributed to the changing lever arm and the difficulty of maintaining the alignment of the shoulder joint axis of rotation with the axis of rotation of the machine. Using smaller ROM may be more appropriate (0 to 90 degrees) for shoulder flexion and abduction during eccentric isokinetic exercise.

Tables 6-3 and 6-4 highlight eccentric isokinetic protocols used for testing and training internal and external rotators in nonsurgical and surgical shoulder patients.

Table 6-3. Sorensen Eccentric Isokinetic Programs for the Shoulder Rotators in Nonsurgical Diagnoses.

Diagnosis	Muscle Group	Program Progression	Special Precautions
Tendonitis, bursitis, impingement syndrome	Internal and external rotators	Initially 2–3 sets of 10 reps at 30°/s Gradual progression to 60°, 90°, 120°, 150°/s Up to 180°/s in athletes 90 reps maximum per session	Painfree ROM Midflexion position preferred Train in nonacute phase
Anterior dislocation	Internal rotators	Use concentric/eccentric mode Initially 2–3 sets of 10 reps at 30°/s Progress to 30°, 60°, 90°/s (3 sets of 10 each) May advance to speeds up to 150°/s and 180°/s in athletes 90 reps maximum per session	Painfree ROM Midflexion position preferred Begin training 6–12 weeks postdislocation Manually palpate the shoulder during training to ensure shoulder stability

Abbreviation: ROM, range of motion.

Nonsurgical Diagnoses

Most nonsurgical shoulder patients benefit from internal and external rotation activities for strengthening the rotator cuff musculature. A progression of positions is effective for initial safety and gradual increase to more difficult activity. Modifying the traditional shoulder isokinetic positions by keeping the humerus below 90 degrees of abduction is recommended to reduce the risk of injury. Elevation of the arm above 90 degrees of flexion or abduction has been shown to develop high intramuscular pressure with resulting muscle ischemia.[55] The midflexion and midabduction shoulder positions in sitting or standing are preferred over the traditional position for initial training of the shoulder internal and external rotators, especially during eccentric isokinetic training

Table 6-4. Sorensen Eccentric Isokinetic Programs for the Shoulder Rotators in Surgical Cases

Diagnosis	Program Progression	Special Precautions
Arthroscopic surgery for debridement of rotator cuff tendons, removal of torn labrum, acromioplasty	Concentric/eccentric mode for both internal and external rotation Initially 2–3 sets of 10 reps at 30°/s with gradual progression to 60°, 90°, 120°, and 150°/s Up to 180°/s in athletes	Consult physician Begin when patient has 80% of full ROM, usually 4–6 weeks postop Midflexion position preferred 90 reps maximum per session
Capsulorraphy[56]	Similar to above	Consult physician Begin when patient has 80% of full ROM for flexion, abduction, and internal rotation, usually 2 to 3 weeks postop Use painfree ROM
Acromioplasty and clavicular resection with or without rotator cuff repair	Initially 2–3 sets of 10 reps at 30°/s and advance to a new speed each week. Work up to 3 sets of 10 reps at 30°, 60°, and 90°/s 90 reps maximum per session Advanced patients may progress up to 150°/s and up to 180°/s for athletes	Consult physician Rotator cuff repair-resistive work begins after 8 weeks. Average is 10–12 weeks postop for concentric/eccentric work Without rotator cuff repair resistive work begins after 6 weeks. Average is 8–10 weeks postop for concentric/eccentric work

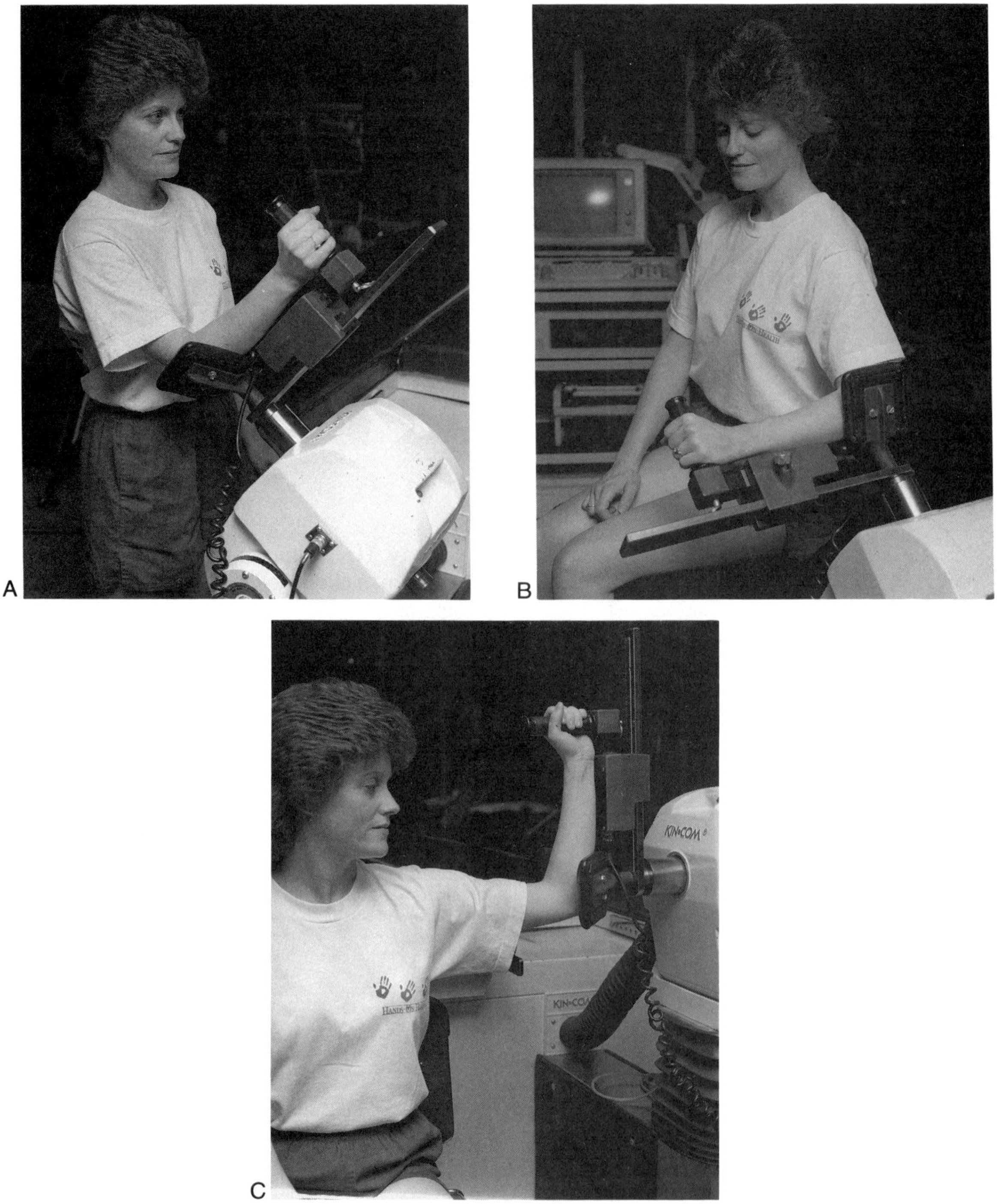

Fig. 6-12. (A) Midflexion position. Subject sitting or standing beside the dynamometer with the tested extremity at 0 degree glenohumeral abduction, 45 degrees of glenohumeral flexion, and 90 degrees of elbow flexion. **(B)** Midabduction position. Subject sitting or standing with the tested extemity at 45 degree glenohumeral abduction, 0 degree of glenohumeral flexion, and 90 degrees of elbow flexion. **(C)** Traditional position. Subject sitting or standing with the tested extremity at 90 degrees glenohumeral abduction, 0 degree of glenohumeral flexion, and 90 degrees of elbow flexion.

(Fig. 6-12). All eccentric isokinetics for the shoulder patient should be performed in the nonpainful range.

Tendonitis, Bursitis, Impingement Syndrome

Focusing on the rotator cuff musculature through positions of midflexion progressing to midabduction is recommended for patients in the nonacute phase. Initiate exercise with 3 sets of 10 repetitions at 30 degrees per second. The recommended progression of activity is listed in Table 6-3. A gradual increase in repetitions to a maximum number of 90 repetitions is recommended per session.

Anterior Dislocation

Palpation of the shoulder during movement is advised to check for joint stability and to insure proper movement of the humerus in the glenohumeral joint. For safety, most training is recommended in the midflexion position.

Surgical Procedures

Consulting with the physician is recommended prior to initiating eccentric isokinetics for all patients. The guidelines listed are general and the concepts and philosophies for rehabilitation may vary regionally.

Arthroscopic Surgery

Patients having arthroscopic surgery for debridement of rotator cuff tendons, removal of the torn labrum, or acromioplasty may begin eccentric isokinetics when the patient achieves 80 percent of full shoulder ROM in flexion, abduction, and rotation, usually 4 weeks postoperatively.

Capsulorraphy

Following the repair of the anterior capsule with a staple for anterior instability, eccentric isokinetic training may follow the guidelines listed for general shoulder arthroscopic surgery; however, eccentric isokinetics should be restricted for internal rotation initially in the midflexion or midabduction positions using a limited range of 30 to 90 degrees.[56] Depending on the approval of the physician, eccentric isokinetics for the external rotators may be performed approximately 4 weeks postoperatively. Palpation of the shoulder during activity is important to confirm proper joint movement (Fig. 6-13). Figure 6-14 shows examples of the isokinetic concentric and eccentric force produced by the shoulder internal and external rotators in a patient 1 year following a capsulorraphy.

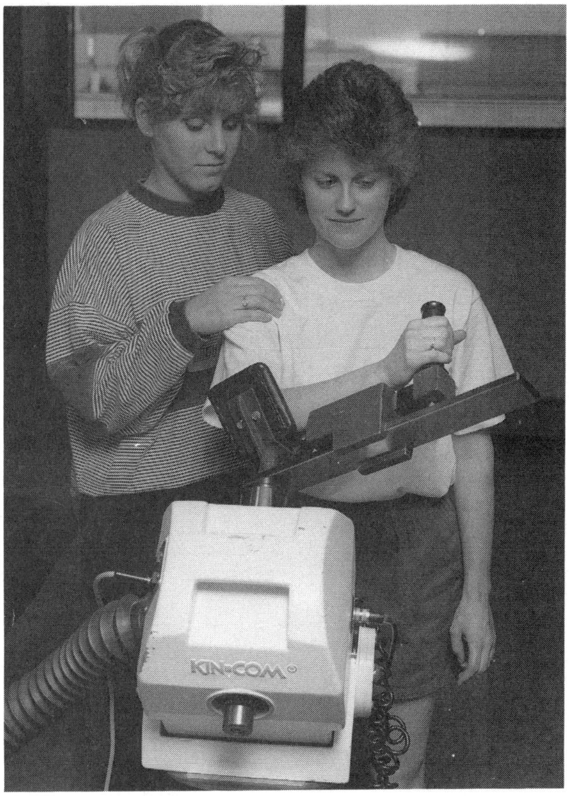

Fig. 6-13. Therapist palpating the glenohumeral joint prior to and during eccentric isokinetic activity to confirm joint stability.

Acromioplasty and Clavicular Resection

The average individual would begin eccentric isokinetic training at 8 weeks following guidelines listed for arthroscopic surgical patients. If the surgery includes repair of the supraspinatus, the average individual would be ready for eccentric isokinetics at 10 to 12 weeks postoperatively.

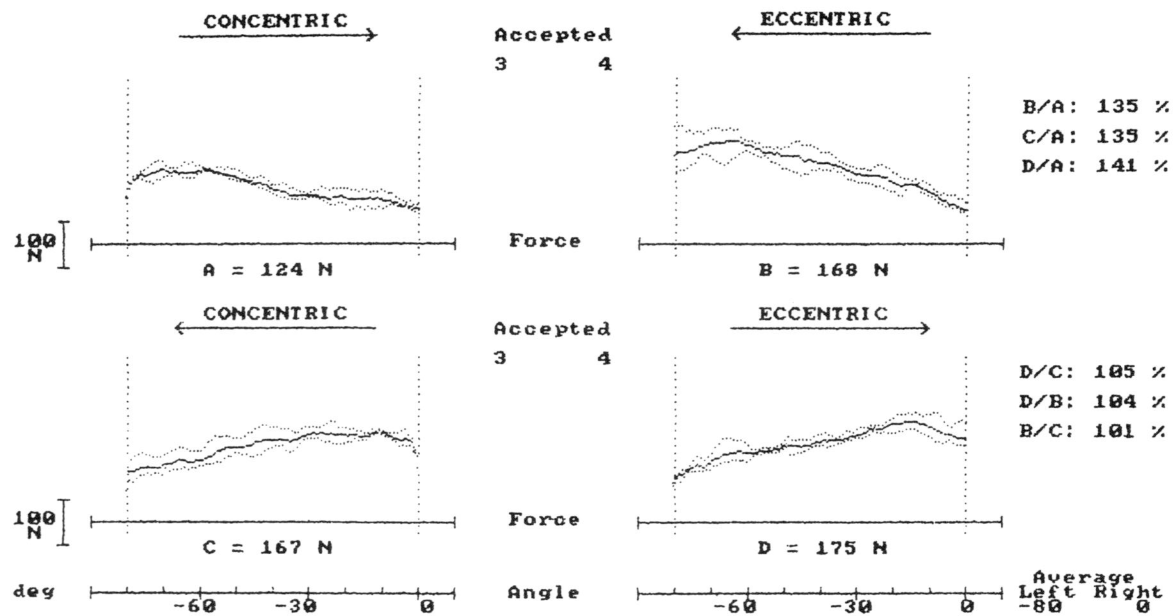

Remarks : LEFT EXTERNAL ROTATORS TESTED 35% STRONGER THAN RIGHT CONCENTRICALLY.
LEFT EXTERNAL ROTATORS TESTED 04% STRONGER THAN RIGHT ECCENTRICALLY.

A

Fig. 6-14. Kin-Com force curves of **(A)** the shoulder external rotators and **(B)** the shoulder internal rotators at 30 degrees per second in a 25-year-old patient, 1 year following a capsulorraphy. *A*, concentric average force produced by the injured limb; *B*, eccentric average force produced by the injured limb; *C*, concentric average force produced by the uninjured limb; *D*, eccentric average force produced by the uninjured limb. (*Figure continues.*)

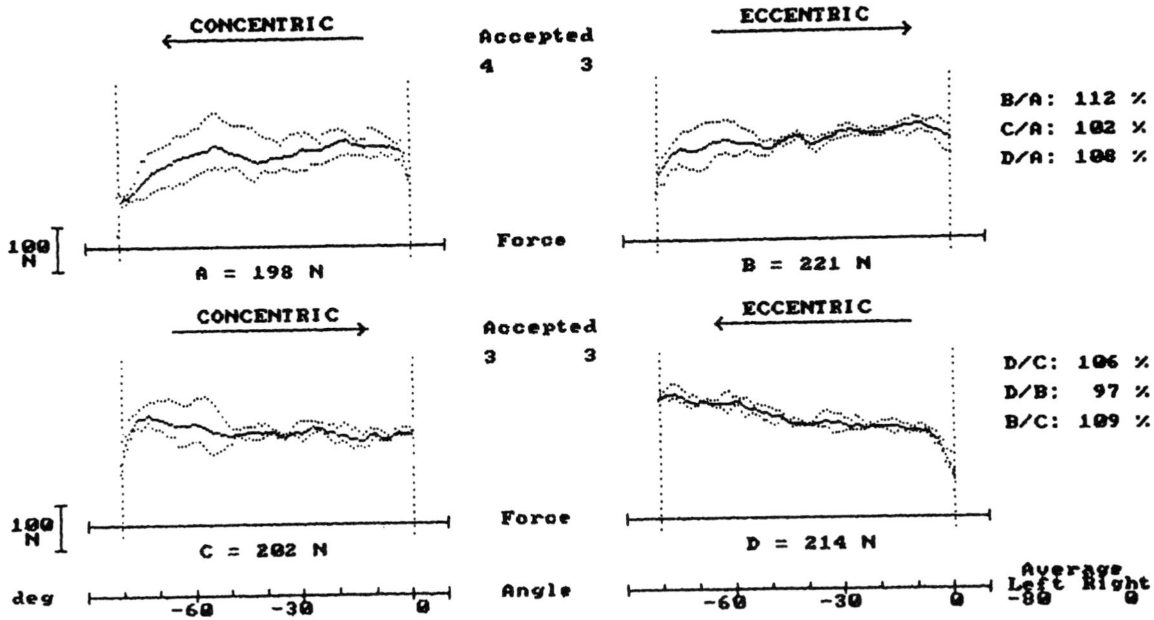

Remarks : LEFT INTERNAL ROTATORS TESTED 02% STRONGER THAN RIGHT CONCENTRICALLY.

B DEFICIENCY OF INTERNAL ROTATORS LEFT ECCENTRICALLY=03%

Fig. 6-14 *(Continued)*.

A

B

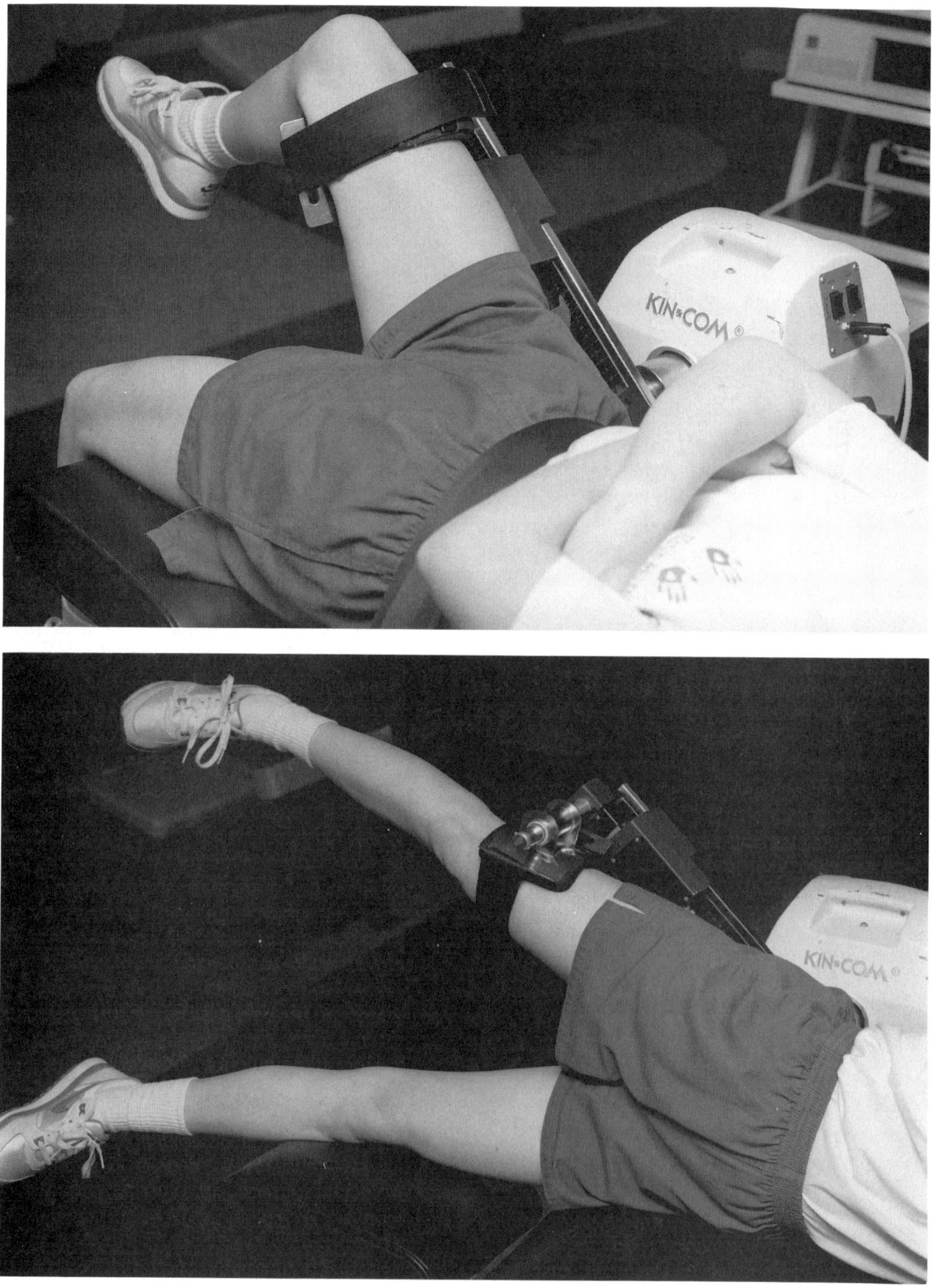

Fig. 6-15. Positioning used for **(A)** hip extension and **(B)** hip abduction eccentric isokinetic testing.

OTHER JOINT TESTING

Various pathologies and injuries other than those relating to the knee or shoulder may benefit from eccentric isokinetic exercise although documentation of rehabilitation programs for other joints is not readily available. Isokinetic devices accommodate to eccentric training of the hip and ankle. The guidelines for training these areas are similar to those for the knee. Eccentric isokinetic exercise may be added to the rehabilitation program when effusion, ROM, and pain permit in the nonacute phase. Begin at the slower speeds with 3 sets of 10 repetitions at 30 degrees per second in the painfree ROM. The program may be progressed to 3 sets of 10 repetitions at speeds of 60, 90, and 120 degrees per second for a total of 90 repetitions maximum per session. Athletes tolerate up to 180 degrees per second.

Positioning and stabilization are problems observed clinically when testing the hip. When testing hip abductors and hip extensors in 12 amateur ice hockey players, verbal cues were needed to maintain the positioning despite using stabilization straps (Sorenson and Gross, unpublished data, 1989). The hockey players were positioned on their sides for hip abduction and supine for hip extension (Fig. 6-15). When using a bilateral comparison, deficits of less than 10 percent were observed in that population.

Positioning of the ankle joint is difficult because of its complex axis of rotation and the difficulty matching the joint axis of rotation with the machine axis of rotation. Positioning of the ankle has been shown to effect torque.[57] Manufacturers are continually upgrading all attachments to improve the stabilization and alignment. Examples of positioning for ankle eccentric isokinetic testing are included on Figure 6-16.

Eccentric isokinetic training is appropriate for training patients with recurrent ankle sprains. Clifford and Voight introduce eccentric isokinetics

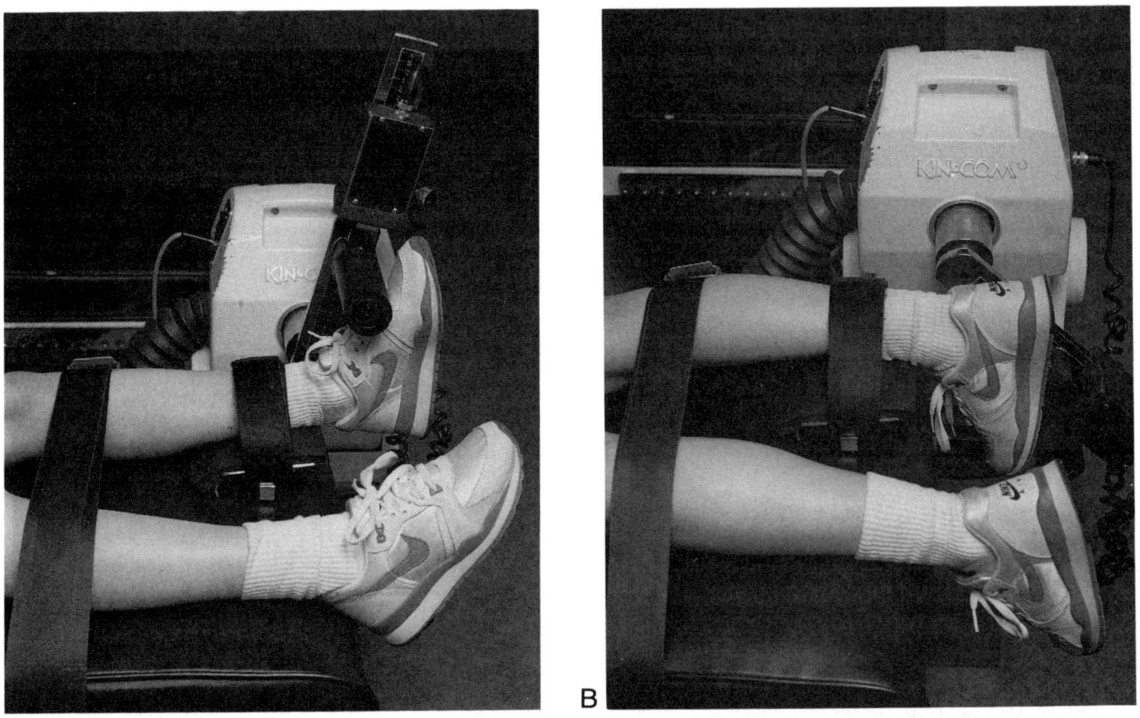

A B

Fig. 6-16. Position used for **(A)** ankle dorsiflexion and **(B)** ankle plantar flexion isokinetic testing on the Kin-Com. **(C)** Position used for ankle plantar flexion and dorsiflexion testing on the Biodex. (*Figure continues.*)

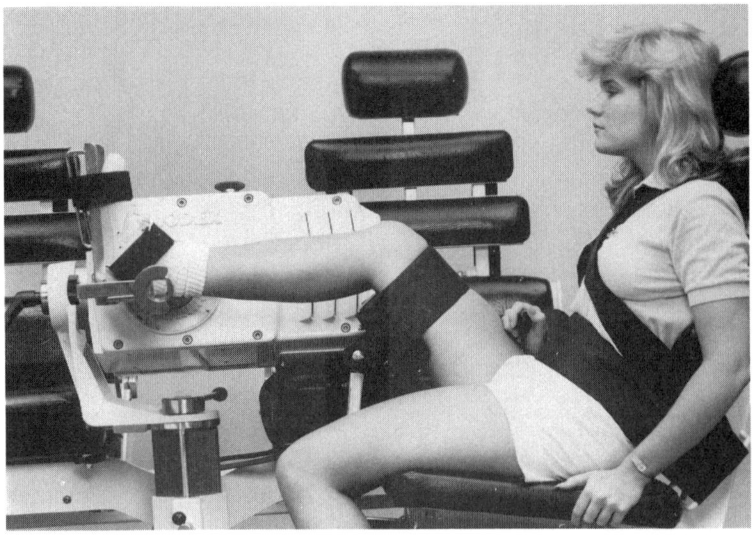

C

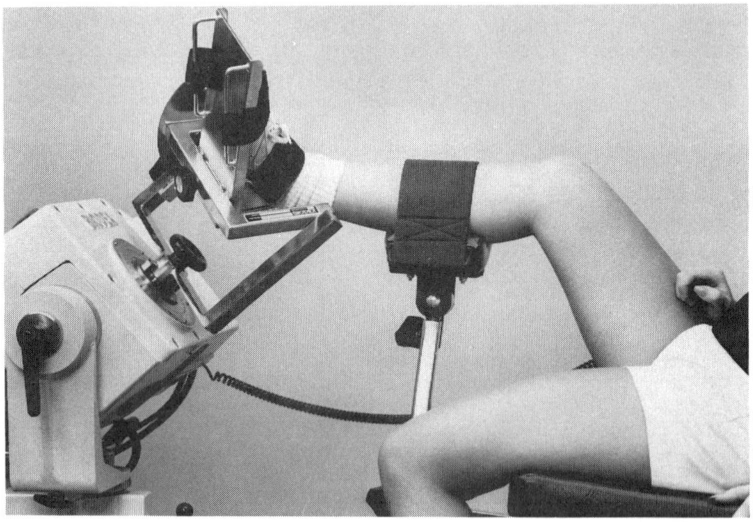

D

Fig. 6-16 (*Continued*). **(D)** Position used for ankle inversion and eversion testing on the Biodex. (Figs. C and D from Biodex Operators Manual,[62] with permission.)

when the patient can walk without pain and when the swelling is under control.[58] They introduce the patients at 30 degrees per second in the passive mode encouraging concentric and eccentric contractions of the peroneals. As long as the patient remains painfree the speed is increased to 120 to 180 degrees per second. Clifford and Voight feel that the value of the data decreases above 180 degrees per second.[58] They reason that exercising over a short arc of motion, the patients expend considerable energy keeping up with the system and are unable to generate significant torque.

Training for the elbow and wrist often follow similar protocols. An example of positioning for eccentric forearm training is displayed in Figure 6-17. Griffen[28] used a threshold of 20 newtons

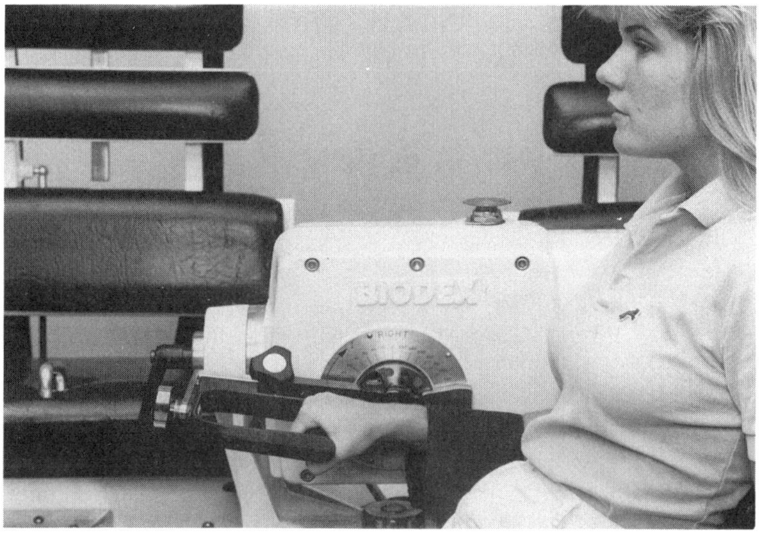

Fig. 6-17. Positioning for wrist flexion/extension testing using the Biodex. (From Biodex Operators Manual,[62] with permission.)

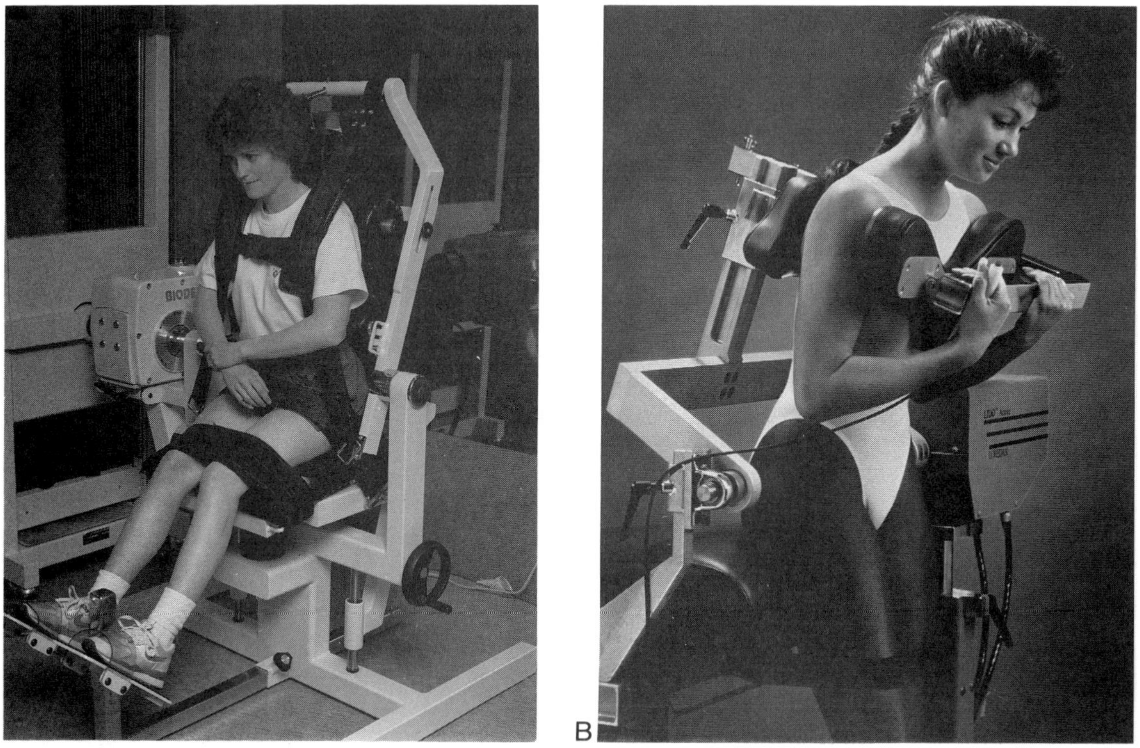

A B

Fig. 6-18. Positioning for trunk testing and training using **(A)** the Biodex and **(B)** the Lido. Positioning for trunk testing and training using the LIDO. (Courtesy of Loredan, Davis, CA.)

when testing the elbow flexors eccentrically in 30 healthy women. She tested at zero, 30, 120, and 210 degrees per second but found low test-retest reliability.

Devices are available for eccentric testing and training of the trunk musculature and this type of training is growing in popularity (Fig. 6-18). Formal protocols have not been developed. Dr. Rowinski in the Biodex Clinical Protocol manual suggests that isokinetic exercise of the trunk should progress from eccentrics of the trunk extensors, to concentrics of the flexors, and finally to concentrics of the trunk extensors.[59] A protocol used by Nix and Clemmer[60] use eccentric isokinetics as part of their comprehensive back program. Initial workouts consist of concentric and eccentric contractions using the passive mode at 30 degrees per second progressing to 60 and 90 degrees per second.

TESTING

Eccentric testing procedures for upper and lower extremities should follow the general orientation guidelines. Bilateral comparisons are commonly performed. Formal testing generally involves testing until three reproducible maximal contractions are obtained. The testing programs of most devices involve either reciprocal concentric then eccentric testing of a single muscle group, or eccentric testing of agonist to antagonist. Most testing of nonsurgical related diagnoses occurs prior to and post rehabilitation, although the pretest may not be performed due to pain, effusion, or limited ROM. The majority of testing is performed at 30 degrees per second, but may occur at speeds up to 180 degrees per second depending on the time of testing and the patient situation.

GENERAL TRAINING IN HEALTHY POPULATIONS

Specific programs for eccentric isokinetic training in healthy populations are not published. It is possible that eccentric isokinetic training may enhance functional or athletic performance; however, research is needed to determine the value of eccentric isokinetic training as well as optimal training methods. The cost of eccentric isokinetic training will most likely limit its use for healthy populations, with the possible exception of use by professional athletes.

SUMMARY

Eccentric isokinetic testing and training contributes to the overall rehabilitation of an individual because eccentric muscular contractions play a major role in functional activities and athletics. Eccentric isokinetic activity differs from concentric isokinetic activity in the production of force at a specific angle and in the force-velocity relationship. Although eccentric torque has been found to increase as velocity increases, it remains unclear whether this increase places an individual at greater risk for injury. Most research indicates that the torque production at faster speeds tends to plateau.

Eccentric isokinetic testing and training may be safely performed if several precautions are followed. The timing which eccentric isokinetic activity is introduced is crucial as this type of training should not be initiated during the acute phase of injury. Proper orientation and a gradual progression of a program are important.

Further research is needed in many areas of eccentric isokinetic training. Reliability studies should focus on speeds and positions of numerous joints. The force-velocity relationship needs to be identified over a spectrum of velocities and for many muscle groups. Research on the effects of eccentric isokinetic activity in clinical populations would be helpful in the development of training programs.

It is important for the clinician to use eccentric isokinetics as an adjunct to a rehabilitation program. Sound clinical judgement should be followed when implementing eccentric isokinetic activity to insure both safety and success.

REFERENCES

1. Ellenbecker TS, Davies GJ, Rowinski MJ: Concentric versus eccentric isokinetic strengthening of the rotator cuff: Objective data versus functional test. Am J Sports Med 16:64, 1988

2. Winter DA: Movements of force and mechanical power in jogging. J Biomech 16:91, 1983
3. Abrahams WH: Exercise induced muscle soreness. Phys Sports Med 12:94, 1980
4. Thorstensson A, Karlsson J: Fatiguability and fibre composition of human skeletal muscle. Acta Physiol Scand 98:318, 1976
5. Fleising G: Throwing Analysis. Presentation at the 1990 Injuries in Baseball Course: Medical and Scientific Aspects of Baseball. Birmingham, AL, January 26, 1990
6. Lamb RL: Manual muscle testing. p. 47. In Rothstein JM (ed): Measurement in Physical Therapy. Churchill Livingstone, New York, 1985
7. Lankhorst GJ, Van de Stadt RJ, Van der Korst JK: The relationships of functional capacity, pain, and isometric and isokinetic torque in osteoarthrosis of the knee. Scand J Rehabil Med 17:167, 1985
8. Mayhew TP, Rothstein JM: Measurement of Muscle performance with instruments. p. 57. In Rothstein JM (ed): Measurement in Physical Therapy. Churchill Livingstone, New York, 1985
9. Rothstein JM, Lamb, RL, Mayhew TP: Clinical uses of isokinetic measurements: Critical issues. Phys Ther 67:1840, 1988
10. Grace TG, Sweetster ER, Nelson MA, et al: Isokinetic muscle imbalance and knee joint injuries. J Bone Joint Surg 66A:734, 1984
11. Hageman PA, Gillaspie DM, Hill LD: Effects of speed and limb dominance on eccentric and concentric isokinetic testing of the knee. J Ortho Sports Phys Ther 10:59, 1988
12. Lucca JA, Kline KK: Effects of upper and lower limb preference on torque production in the knee flexors and extensors. J Orthop Sports Phys Ther 11:202, 1989
13. Cook EE, Gray VL, Savinar-Nogue E, Medeiros J: Shoulder antagonistic strength ratios: A comparison between college-level baseball pitchers and nonpitchers. J Orthop Sports Phys Ther 8:451, 1987
14. Perrin DH, Robertson RJ, Ray RL: Bilateral isokinetic peak torque, torque acceleration energy, power, and work relationship in athletes and nonathletes. J Orthop Sports Phys Ther 9:184, 1987
15. Nosse LJ: Assessment of selected reports on the stength relationship of the knee musculature. J Orthop Sports Phys Ther 4:78, 1982
16. Bennett JG, Stauber WT: Evaluation and treatment of anterior knee pain using eccentric exercise. Med Sci Sports Exerc 18:526, 1986
17. Trudelle-Jackson E, Meske N, Highgenboten C, Jackson C: Eccentric/concentric torque deficits in the quadriceps muscle. J Orthop Sports Phys 'Ther 11:142, 1982
18. Moffroid M, Whipple R, Hofkosh J et al: A study of isokinetic exercise. Phys Ther 49:735, 1969
19. Farrell M, Richards JF: Analysis of the reliability and validity of the kinetic communicator exercise device. Med Sci Sports Exerc 18:44, 1986
20. Hanten WP, Lange JC: Reliability and validity of the kinetic communicator for the measurements of torque, work, and power. Phys Ther 68:825, 1988
21. Rothstein JM: Measurement and clinical practice: Theory and application. p. 1. In Rothstein JM (ed): Measurement in Physical Therapy. Churchill Livingstone, New York, 1985
22. Taylor RL, Casey JJ: Quadriceps torque production on the Cybex II dynamometer as related to changes in lever arm length. J Orthop Sports Phys Ther 8:147, 1986
23. Bottjen E, Batterton T, Ehrich K et al: Effects of stationary and nonstationary input cuffs on peak torque measurements. Phys Ther 69:378, 1989
24. Jackson A, Highgenboten C, Meske N, Trudelle-Jackson E: Univariate and multivariate analysis of the reliability of the kinetic communicator. Med Sci Sports Exerc, suppl. 19:23, 1987
25. Snow CJ, Johnson K: Reliability of two velocity-controlled tests for the measurement of peak torque of the knee flexors during resisted muscle shortening and resisted muscle lengthening. Phys Ther 68:781, 1988
26. Wessel J, Mattison G, Luongo F, Isherwood L: Reliability of eccentric and concentric measurements. Phys Ther 68:782, 1988
27. Wilhite MR, Cohen ER, Wilhite SC: Reliability of concentric and eccentric measurement of the quadriceps performance using the KIN-COM dynamometer: The effect of testing order for three different speeds. J Orthop Sports Phys Ther 11:419, 1990
28. Griffen JW: Differences in elbow flexion torque measured concentrically, eccentrically, and isometrically. Phys Ther 67:1205, 1987
29. Hageman PA, Gillaspie DK, Hill LD: Effects of position and speed on eccentric and concentric isokinetic testing of the shoulder rotators. J Orthop Sports Phys Ther 11:64, 1989
30. Appen L, Duncan PW: Strength relationship of the knee musculature: Effects of gravity and sport. J Orthop Sports Phys Ther 7:232, 1986
31. Fillyaw M, Berins T, Fernandez L: Importance of correcting isokinetic peak torque for the effect of gravity when calculating knee flexor to extensor muscle ratios. Phys Ther 66:23, 1986

32. Figoni SF, Christ CB, Massey BH: Effects of speed, hip and knee angle, and gravity on hamstring to quadriceps torque ratios. J Orthop Sports Phys Ther 9:287, 1988
33. Francis K, Hoobler T: Comparison of peak torque values of the knee flexor and extensor muscle groups using the Cybex II and Lido 2.0 isokinetic dynamometers. J Orthop Sports Phys Ther 8:480, 1987
34. Wilk KE, Johnson RD, Levine B: A comparison of peak torque values of knee extension and flexor muscle groups using Biodex, Cybex, and KIN-COM isokinetic dynamometers. Phys Ther 68:792, 1988
35. Timm K: Comparison of knee extensor and flexor muscle group performances using the Cybex 340 and the MERAC isokinetic dynamometer. Phys Ther 69:389, 1989
36. Rodgers KL, Berger RA: Motor-unit involvement and tension during maximal, voluntary concentric, eccentric, and isometric contractions of the elbow flexors. Med Sci Sports Exerc 6:253, 1974
37. Walmsley RP, Pearson N, Stymiest P: Eccentric wrist extensor contractions and the force velocity relationship in muscle. J Orthop Sports Phys Ther 8:288, 1986
38. Hanten W, Wieding D: Isokinetic measurement of the force-velocity relationship of concentric and eccentric contractions. Phys Ther 68:801, 1988
39. Chandler JM, Duncan PW: Eccentric vs. concentric force-velocity relationships of the quadriceps femoris muscle. Phys Ther 68:800, 1988
40. Eloranto V, Komi PV: Function of the quadriceps femoris muscle under maximal concentric and eccentric contractions. Electromyogr Clin Neurophysiol 20:159, 1980
41. Bohannon RW, Gajodsik RL, LeVeau BF: Isokinetic knee flexion and extension torque in the upright sitting and semireclined sitting positions. Phys Ther 66:1083, 1986
42. Barr EA, Duncan PW: Influence of position on knee flexor peak torque. J Orthop Sports Phys Ther 9:279, 1988
43. Charteris J, Goslin G: The effects of position and movement velocity on isokinetic force output at the knee. J Sports Med 22:154, 1982
44. Soderberg GJ, Blaschak MJ: Shoulder internal and external rotation peak torque production through a velocity spectrum in differing positions. J Orthop Sports Phys Ther 8:518, 1987
45. Walmsley RP, Szybbo C: A comparative study of the torque generated by the shoulder internal and external rotator muscles in different positions and at varying speeds. J Orthop Sports Phys Ther 9:217, 1987
46. Hay JG, Feuerbach JW: The effects of concentric training on eccentric strength. Contemporary PT 1 (1):1, 4, 1988-1989
47. Nicely K, Schultz C, Porter S et al: Effects of training using isokinetic-concentric, isokinetic-concentric, and isometric contractions on the peak torque of the knee extensors. Phys Ther 68:799, 1988
48. McCurry D, Davies GJ, Rowinski MJ et al: Effects of a Seven-Week Isokinetic Training Program on Eccentric Strength Development. Med Sci Sports Exerc, suppl. 19:S7, 1986
49. Komi PV, Viitasalo JT: Changes in motor unit activity and metabolism in human skeletal muscle during and after repeated eccentric and concentric contractions. Acta Physiol Scand 100:246, 1977
50. Komi PV, Rusko H: Quantitative evaluation of mechanical and electrical changes during fatigue loading of eccentric and concentric work. Scand J Rehabil Med, suppl. 3:S121, 1974
51. Gray JC, Chandler JM: Percent decline in peak torque production during repeated concentric and eccentric contractions of the quadriceps femoris muscle. J Orthop Sports Phys Ther 11:309, 1989
52. DeNuccio DK, Davies GJ, Rowinski MJ: Comparison of quadriceps isokinetic eccentric and isokinetic concentric data using a standard fatigue protocol. Phys Ther 66:794, 1986
53. Jenson K, DiFabio RP: Evaluation of eccentric exercise in treatment of patellar tendonitis. Phys Ther 69:211, 1989
54. Indelicato PA, Huegel M: The anterior cruciate ligament: ACL rupture with medial and lateral meniscal damage. In Biodex Clinical Application Manual. Biodex Corp, Shirley, NY, 1988
55. Jarvholm U, Palmerud G, Styf J et al: Intramuscular pressure in the supraspinatus muscle. J Orthop Res 6:230, 1988
56. Gross RM: Artheroscopic shoulder capsulorraphy: Does it work? Am J Sports Med 17:495, 1989
57. Oberg B, Bergman T, Tropp H: Testing of isokinetic muscle strength in the ankle. Med Sci Sports Exerc 19:318, 1987
58. Clifford SJ, Voight M: Ankle injury: Third degree sprain of lateral collateral ligaments. In Biodex Clinical Application Manual. Biodex Corp, Shirley, NY, 1988
59. Rowinski M: Biodex Operation Manual. Biodex Corp, Shirley, NY, 1989

60. Nix JE, Clemmer D: Low back pain: Ruptured lumbar disk with internal disk disruption. In Biodex Clinical Application Manual. Biodex Corp, Shirley, NY, 1989
61. Morrissey MC: The relationship between peak torque and work of the quadriceps and hamstrings after a meniscectomy. J Orthop Sports Phys Ther 8:405, 1987
62. Biodex Operator's Manual, Biodex Corp, Shirley, NY

7

Free Weight Training

MARK ALBERT
JIM LATHROP

Dedicated to the memory of Dave Pasanella (1962–1990). World record holder power lifting, heavyweight class; "World's Strongest Man"; all-time records: squat, 1030.2 lb; 3 lift total, 2,458 lb. Strength and conditioning coach, Georgia Tech Athletic Association, Atlanta, GA, 1985–1990

PHILOSOPHY STATEMENT

Strength and power training with weights, whether free plates with bars or weight stack machines; are traditional forms of applying the eccentric loading principles described in previous chapters. The purpose of this chapter is to provide a practical overview of successful and effective free weight training lifts, review major safety and injury prevention considerations, and describe timing and weight guidelines in a year-round program design. While the popularity of free weights in many disciplines and varied sports has increased dramatically in the past decade, our approach will involve a generic structuring of various lifts to provide overall performance training success, injury prevention, and specific skills in selected lifts.

The concept of strength training has asssumed new importance in all explosive and team-oriented sports, due to the competitive pressures in today's society. Both male and female athletes have recognized the performance advantages associated with increased muscular strength and power, increased lean body mass and in some cases, increased body weight can transfer into potential for greater momentum. In addition, because of the selective loading of connective tissues associated with eccentrics, free weights and machines also provide an important measure of injury prevention to joints and tendons. Greater muscle bulk (hypertrophy) coupled with the aforementioned joint structural changes provide a useful protective system against the common compressive forces and direct impacts encountered in many sports settings.

Weight training is a type of eccentric biased training that produces rapid adaptations in the neuromuscular system. Synchronization, or improved neuromuscular recruitment and activation, produces consistent and early changes in strength that are unrelated to actual muscle size increases.[1,2]

Many traditional, popular beliefs about free weight use are being disproved as scientific investigation and clinical trials are reported in the literature. One such belief, that free weight training produces postural deformities and inflexible muscles leading to the so-called "muscle bound" profile, has been shown to be invalid, provided the athlete also practices routine and appropriate flexibility programs in conjunction with the strength/power training. Another popular belief is that heavy weight work in the dead lift and squat lift, (intrinsic to power lifting—see the *Weight*

Authors' note: During the preparation of this chapter, Dave was tragically killed in an auto accident. He will be missed by the many that he helped and his friends and family. I am honored to complete the chapter on his behalf.

Training Principles section), is inherently dangerous to the lumbosacral spine and predisposes an athlete to chronic pathology with associated radiographic changes. This belief is challenged by the empirical data that show that competitive power and Olympic lifters rarely have lumbosacral symptoms or radiographic evidence of joint, disc, or ligamentous damage or degeneration.[3] Finally, the common "wisdom" that squats are tantamount to deep knee bends and are injurious to the knee joint has also been challenged recently. The patellofemoral joint has been implicated as being at risk for injury from the squat movement, but again, competitive lifters rarely experience dysfunction of this joint. Another common belief cautions against squat lifts because of the potential for dangerous levels of strain to be imparted to the knee ligaments, specifically the anterior and posterior cruciate ligaments (ACL and PCL, respectively), causing compensatory insufficiency (commonly called "loose knees"). Perhaps the most substantive study to investigate this relationship not only refuted a loosening of ligamentous tissue about the knee, but based on the use of highly reliable and quantified instrumentation (the KT 1000 Knee Ligament Arthrometer, Medmetric Co.), concluded that squat training produced an actual decrease of ligament and joint laxity with respect to the function of the ACL.[4]

A brief background for this chapter involves definitions of several key terms:

Strength, the ability to produce tension
Muscular endurance, the ability to sustain tension over repeated or continuous efforts
Power, the unit of force per unit of time (relates to speed of movement, or explosiveness)

Training with free weights and machines is effective in developing strength, muscular endurance, and power by appropriate management of the key variables in conditioning programs: intensity, frequency, duration, and cycling (rest versus work periods). It is important to define the distinction between two often misused terms: *weightlifting* and *weight training*. Weightlifting refers to the discipline of a series of specific lifts in competitive events, while weight training is more universal as a mechanism for enhancement of performance in many sports, improvement of overall fitness and physical development, and injury prevention.

WEIGHT TRAINING DISCIPLINES

Numerous physical activities and sports incorporate the use of free weights as primary or supplmental methods of conditioning (Table 7-1). With respect to the differentiation between weight lifting and weight training, three major weight lifting sports exist: Olympic lifting, power lifting, and body building. Each sport has distinctive competitive settings, and training for each is markedly different, based on the principle of specificity. Olympic lifting involves two lifts, the *snatch* and the *clean and jerk*. These lifts combine heavy weights with immense speeds in full body, ballistic, closed chain movements that describe plyometric demands. The lifter's technique is critical to competitive success and injury prevention. The lifts are similar in requiring weights to be raised from floor level in an explosive pulling phase, followed by a rapid squat-under movement to place the weight in each lift's specific rack position (Figs. 7-1 and 7-2). Both lifts require maximal muscular power, skill, and speed. Elite Olympic lifters have produced the highest power outputs ever recorded.[5] Strong eccentric muscle recruitment is required of the lower body antigravity musculature (gluteals, quadriceps, gastrosoleus complex), spinal extensors and deltoids, upper trapezuis, and biceps/triceps. Due to strict technical require-

Table 7-1. Disciplines That Use Free Weights

Lifting sports
Olympic
Power
Body building
Performance training
Football
Track and field
Basketball
Wrestling
General fitness/recreation
Circuit training
Rehabilitation

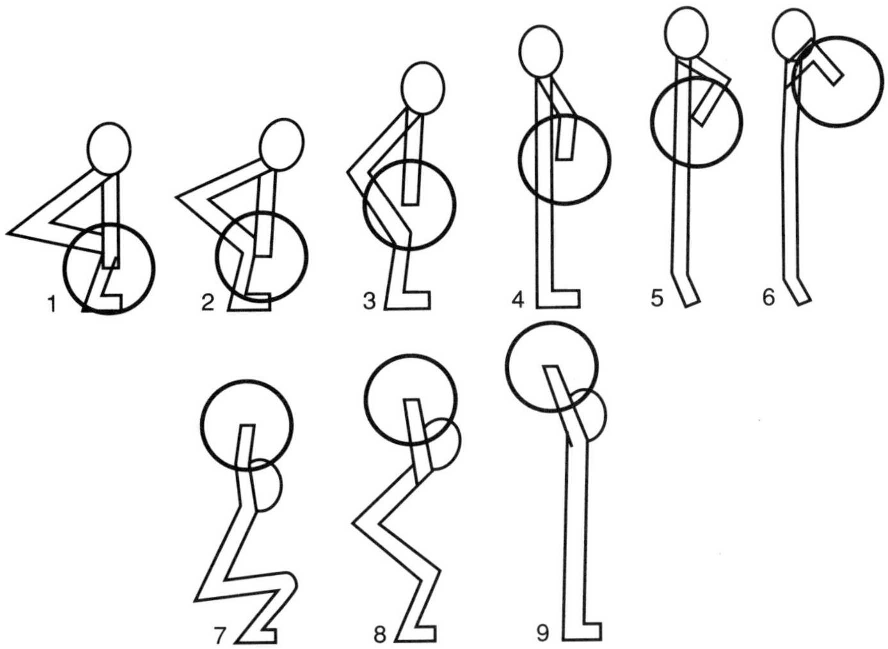

Fig. 7-1. Snatch sequential schematic. (Artwork courtesy of Jerry Albert.)

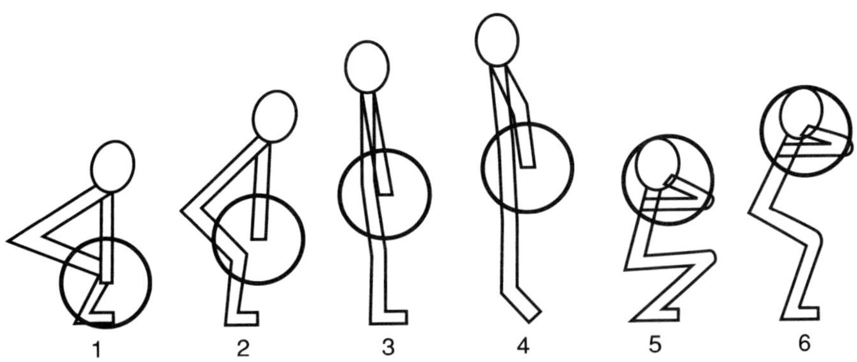

Fig. 7-2. Clean and jerk sequential schematic. (Artwork courtesy of Jerry Albert.)

Table 7-2. Clean and Jerk Technique Checklist

Description of Phases	Point Value
A. Starting stance: head up, back straight, shoulders lightly over bar	0–3
B. Pull: head up, double knee bend, bar close to body, high extension	0–5
C. Clean: quickness, balance, straight back, low squat, elbows high in front, body alignment and balance on stand-up, bar horizontal	0–5
D. Jerk: high arm position, leg drive, split depth and quickness, body alignment and balance on stand-up, bar horizontal	0–7
Total points	0–20

(From Stone and O'Bryant,[19] with permission.)

ments (Tables 7-2 and 7-3), these lifts are less commonly used for weight training applications.

Power lifting is a sport that is popular in the United States and combines three basic lifts in a demanding discipline of sheer, total strength. Power lifters demonstrate massive hypertrophy and low body fat composition. The three lifts practiced by power lifters include the squat, a modification of knee bends; the bench press, probably the best overall expression of upper body strength other than simple grip strength, and the dead lift, which involves raising a weight from the floor to waist level. In competition, the athletes' individual lifts are added to determine meet results, such that total body strength is paramount to success. The component power lifts are routinely used as the basis for many weight and strength training programs for a host of diverse sports.

Table 7-3. Snatch Technique Checklist

Description of Phases	Point Value
A. Starting position: head up, wide grip back straight, shoulders slightly over bar	0–3
B. Pull: head up, double knee bend, bar close to body, high extension	0–7
C. Hop: quickness, balance straight back, low squat, shoulder flexibility	0–7
D. Stand-Up: lateral and forward stability, body alignment, elbows straight, bar horizontal	0–3
Total points	0–20

(From Stone and O'Bryant,[19] with permission.)

The final discipline in free weight lifting involves body building. Body building is devoted to the creation of superior muscular development in a symmetrical and esthetic physique. Competition involves a series of poses with maximal isometric postures to favorably show individual muscle group definition, shape and size. While absolute strength is not a direct goal, body builders must achieve very low body fat levels and training regimens may last many hours to achieve this lean, "cut" look. Body builders primarily use isolated muscle lifts with high repetitions.

SPECIFICS OF POWER LIFTS

Because of the widespread use of power lifts, especially the squat and bench press, in varied settings, and the important eccentric progression contributions of these lifts, we will carefully examine the appropriate biomechanics of each lift. With appropriate developmental increases, and use of correct techniques and prevention measures (see the section *Injury Prevention Principles*), these lifts are also very safe for general use in weight training and end-stage rehabilitation.

Squats

Although widely used in athletic weight training settings, the squat also contributes to the early preparation for plyometrics and is a functional element in many daily activities, such as sitting and rising from a chair, stooping to pick up objects, negotiating stairs, and using the toilet. The squat serves a primary, base exercise from which to build a lower body eccentric biased progression and is readily applicable to the mid to late stages of sports and orthopedic rehabilitation.

The squat lift has been characterized as the "king" of strengthening exercises and as the premier lift in weight training (Pasanella, personal communication, Atlanta, 1988). The squat incorporates elements of balance, proprioception of spinal and lower extremity joints, strength and power aspects of the trunk and lower body musculature, postural control, flexibility, effective breathing mechanics, mental concentration, and a measure of personal psychological confidence and achievement. Several studies indicate the positive relationship between increased strength and positive self-concept, confidence and personal esteem.[6–9] A key element in performing the squat is the ability to do a dynamic, timed anterior pelvic tilt (increased lumbar lordosis) commonly called "breaking of the hips." This skilled, coordinated action requires balance as the knees flex and demands strong stabilization of the pelvis through eccentric action of the biarticular hamstring muscles and cocontraction of the abdominals and lumbar paraspinals/latissimus dorsi to stabilize a fairly erect position of the trunk (Fig. 7-3).

Three variations of the squat are commonly used with specific attention to the placement of the feet, position of the bar on the trunk, and the isolation of particular muscle groups (Table 7-4). In each squat variation, it is imperative to maintain the bar position directly over the instep of the foot. This simple form principle assures that the knees do not pass over the toes in the sagittal plane. This principle is also important in placing the center of gravity of the weight/athlete's body weight combination directly within the base of support. In addition, when the weight is placed vertically over the instep, the position of the tibias relative to the supporting surface is nearly vertical (Fig. 7-4), which promotes decreased strain of both the patellofemoral joint and the ACL. The "breaking of the hips" also produces a weight distribution toward the heels. The two most common errors among inexperienced lifters with the squat are failure to perform the correct pelvic tilt and forcing the knees too far forward over the toes, both of which occur during the descent (negative or eccentric) phase. Other common technical errors are too narrow or too wide of a stance and positioning the bar high on the shoulders during power squats. In most squat lifts the bar should be placed on the upper back in contact with the posterior deltoid muscle and adjacent to the spine of the scapula (Fig. 7-5).

Beyond the obvious usefulness and importance of the squat to weight training programs, functional and biomechanical considerations make the squat equally applicable to mid-to-late stage rehabilitation of many injuries (i.e., knee sprains and lumbosacral strains) and a primary training method to recruit lower extremity eccentric force and neuromuscular control. As mentioned in Chapter 3, precursor training measures include

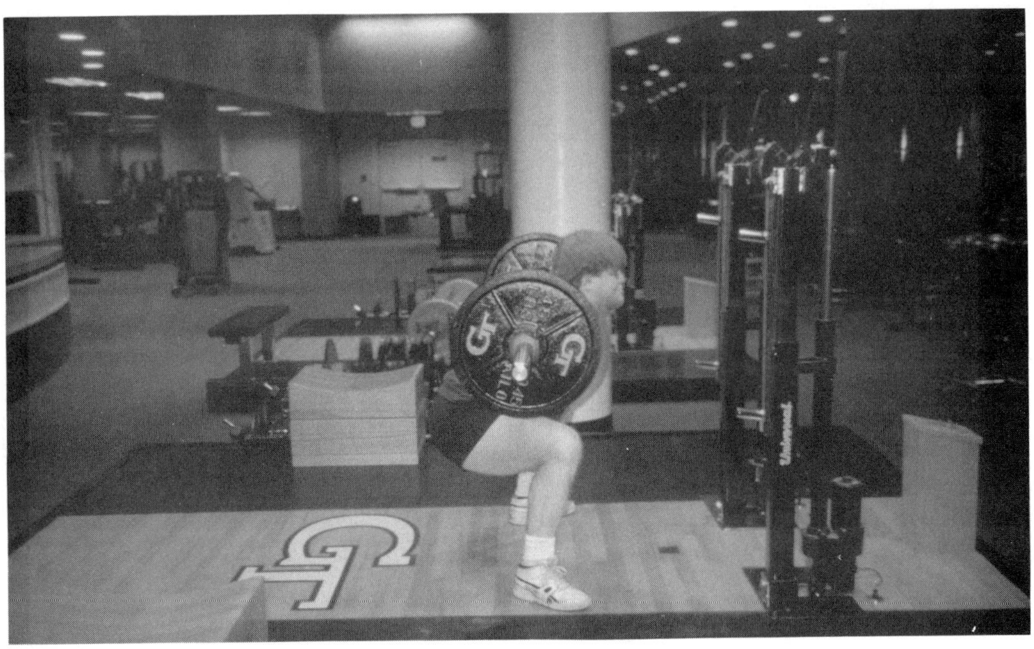

Fig. 7-3. Parallel squat position (thighs parallel to floor).

Table 7-4. Squat Lift Variations

Type of Lift	Base of Support	Bar Position
Front	Feet shoulder width	Bar held at chest
Olympic	Feet wider than shoulders	Bar held high on back
Power	Very wide base	Bar low on shoulders to spine of scapula

basic activities such as step-ups and wall squat slide (back supported against a wall). Increased use of squat progressions in rehabilitation settings is indicated and further research will assist in providing guidelines for optimal use.

Bench Press

A classic challenge and test to upper body strength, the bench press is a popular lift in many fitness and sports settings. The bench press is a compound movement that recruits muscular effort from the anterior deltoid, pectoralis major and minor, and triceps. With technique modifications, it is believed that additional force can be gained from the subscapularis and latissimus dorsi muscles (Pasanella, personal communication, 1988), while stabilization requirements involve the gluteals, lumbar paraspinals, and abdominals. Key technique variations during the lift include hand grip style and width on the bar, pattern of weight ascent and descent, and elbow joint alignment (Table 7-5). Although subject to individual preference, the safest grip style is the overhand grip, whereby the bar rests in the palm with both the fingers and the thumb wrapped completely around it.

Depending on the amount of weight lifted, the athlete should breathe during each repetition to avoid valsalva. Inhalation is performed upon accepting the weight from the stand, while one suggestion for effective exhalation timing is at the so-

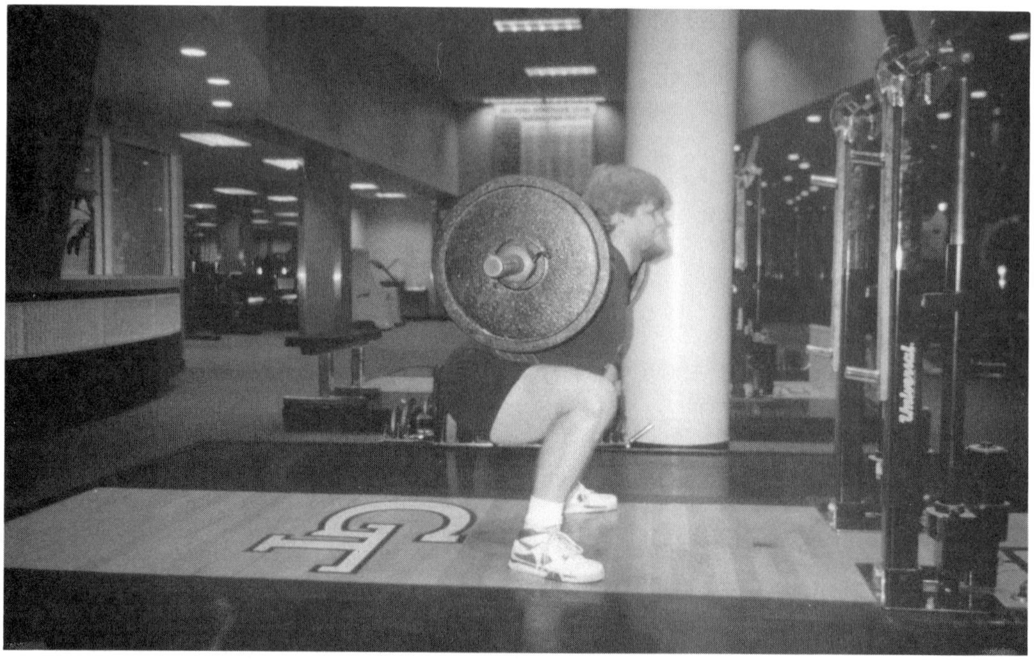

Fig. 7-4. Proper tibial alignment during squat descent.

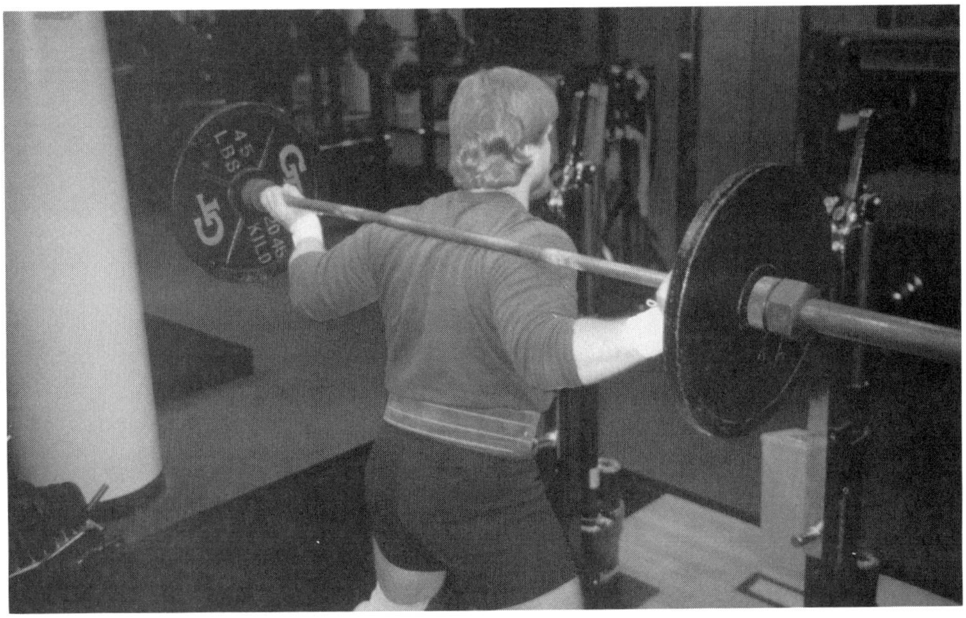

Fig. 7-5. Bar placement position for squat.

called "stick point," presumably when muscle effort changes from predominantly pectoralis muscles to combined triceps/anterior deltoid activity.[10]

When setting up the body position on the bench, it is important to place the head directly under the bar, and firmly plant the feet on the floor. Producing a mild arch to the low back will cause the chest to rise, which will decrease the net mechanical work required of the muscles during the lift. As a result of the grip position on the bar, the elbows should be flexed to approximately 90 degrees when the bar reaches the sternum. Women tend to have less than a 90 degree flexed position, due to a general lack of upper body strength.[10] A wider grip on the bar will effectuate a decrease in the amount of distance between the sternum and the lock-out position of the weight at the completion of the lift.

The bench press is performed in two primary phases: the initial descent phase (immediately after removing the bar from the stand) and the final, ascent phase (Figs. 7-6 and 7-7). The descent phase is primarily eccentric activity of the pectoralis and triceps, with assistive effort from concentric activity of the long head of the biceps brachii. The ascent phase is dominated by concentric activity of the triceps, anterior deltoid, and pectoralis, with stabilization from lumbar and midthoracic paraspinals. It is imperative that the descent phase is performed slowly and smoothly to avoid bouncing on the chest. The injuries that can occur from the bench press (sternal contusion, costochondral stretch and pectoralis rupture) are caused by lack of control during the eccentric, descent phase.

In a contrasting manner, the ascent phase should be performed as explosively as possible to

Table 7-5. Bench Press Variations

Grip Style	Body Orientation	Dominant Muscle Group
Narrow	Shoulder width	Triceps
Medium	Shoulder width to 30″	Triceps/pectorals
Wide	Greater than 30″	Pectorals

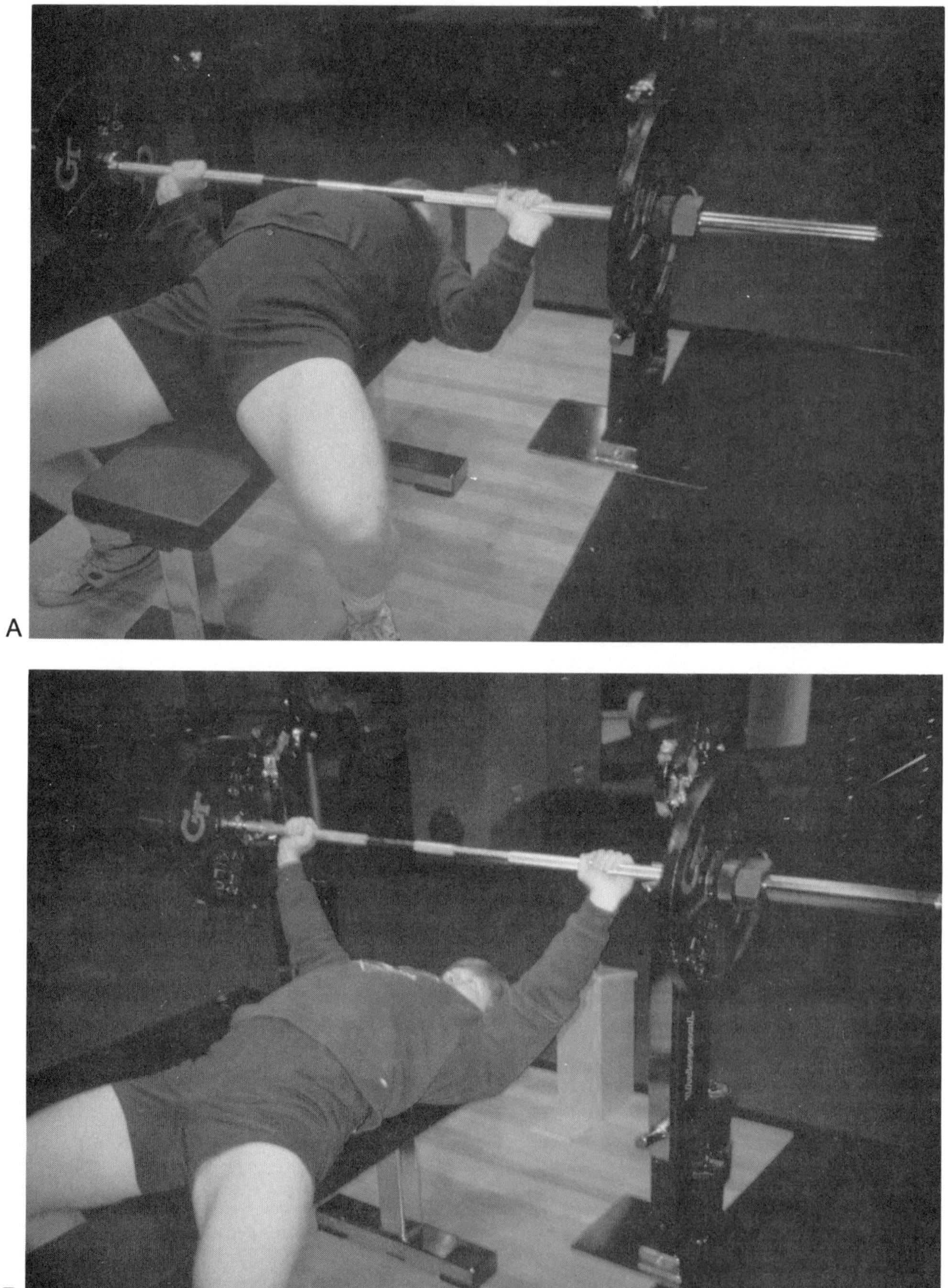

Fig. 7-6. Bench press. **(A)** Ascent phase, beginning position. **(B)** Descent phase, beginning position.

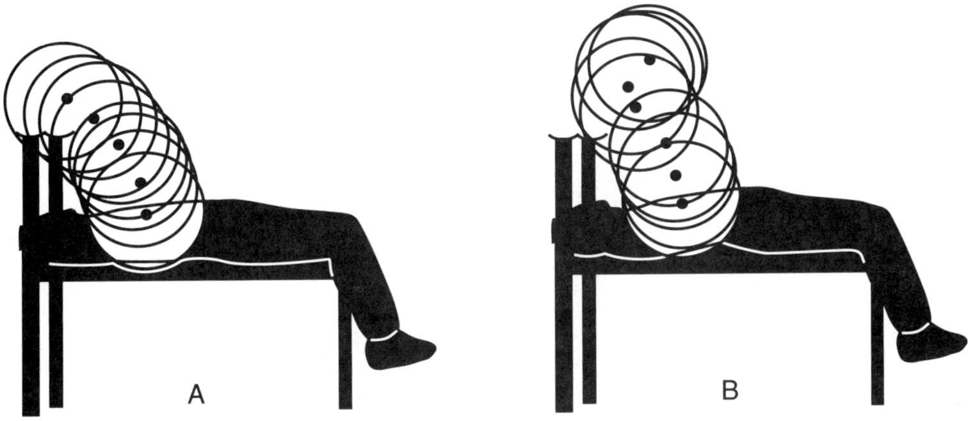

Fig. 7-7. Movement path of bar during bench press. **(A)** Novice. **(B)** Expert. (Artwork courtesy of Jerry Albert.) (Adapted from Stone and O'Bryant,[19] with permission.)

overcome the acceleration of gravity and to recruit the maximal, available muscle fiber. This will minimize the effects of the biomechanical stick point that results at the midphase of the ascent. The same explosive acceleration is also essential during the ascent phase of the squat. Near the completion of the lift it becomes necessary to instantaneously slow the movement to avoid being "thrown" out of safe body alignment.

Dead Lift

The final power lift, the dead lift, may be the ultimate test of raw muscular strength. The lift starts in a forward flexed position of the spine with flexed hips and slight knee flexion, followed by clearing the bar from the floor and uplifting it in one continuous motion until the lifter is standing erect with locked knees (Fig. 7-8). In common with the squat, the dead lift requires maximal effort of the gluteals, hip abductors, and quadriceps with mixed contraction modes of the lumbar extensors and latissimus dorsi. The hamstrings are also maximally recruited in a synergistic eccentric/concentric fashion as they act on the hip and knee simultaneously with corresponding flexibility demands from "toe-touch" like starting and final positions.

The key to a successful, safe lift is a smooth, controlled pull or ascent phase to protect the low back. As with the Olympic lifts, the technical requirements and associated injury potential cause this lift to be infrequently used as a weight training exercise.

Power Clean

Another lift common to weight training programs, the power clean is a variation of the Olympic lifts, with biomechnical similarity to both the squat and the dead lift (Fig. 7-9). Success with this lift combines strength, speed, explosiveness, flexibility, balance, and agility.[11] The versatility of trained skills has made this lift popular in many collegiate weight rooms, especially wth respect to Division 1 football programs.

It is important to maintain an arched back with the head up during this lift and use the hips to provide initial lifting forces. This will cause the arms to remain straight until the weight has reached thigh level, when the shoulders/upper trapezius provide ballistic acceleration to the weight.

Assistance Exercises-Multiple Lifting Exercises

The final area of weight lifting practice involves a series of varied exercises with frec weights and free weight pulley machines or cam-type machines to extend strengthening effects to body areas that are not emphasized in the classic power and/or Olympic lifts. Assistance exercises describe movements that train specific joints and attempt to isolate specific muscles in either open or closed kinetic chains. Assistance exercise training is important to total physical development and is often neglected, leading to muscular imbalances, inferior performance of multijoint lifts, and increased potential for injury.[11] The program composition for assistance exercises is variable and dependent on individual goals and needs; a sample guideline is reviewed in Table 7-6.

Assistance exercises can be used to supplement mass movement patterns or classic free weight lifts, or may constitute a program unto themselves, if power lifts or heavy weights are not desirable, or if the particular needs of a given sport do not require mass movement strength training (i.e., baseball or ballet). The amount of weight used for assistance exercises will vary depending on many intrapersonal variables, however, the heaviest weights that can be controlled with proper form should be used.[11] The great variety of available assistance exercises is demonstrated in a partial listing, grouped according to body area (Table 7-7).

Table 7-6. Assistance Exercise Parameters

Parameters	1 RM (%)	Repetition	Sets
Power	>90	1–3	1–2
Strength	70–90	5–10	2–3
Muscular endurance	60–70	8–12	3

INJURY PREVENTION PRINCIPLES

Optimal success in weightlifting and training is dependent on avoiding injuries. Most injuries associated with weight training/lifting are preventable with the conscientious use of several straight-

A

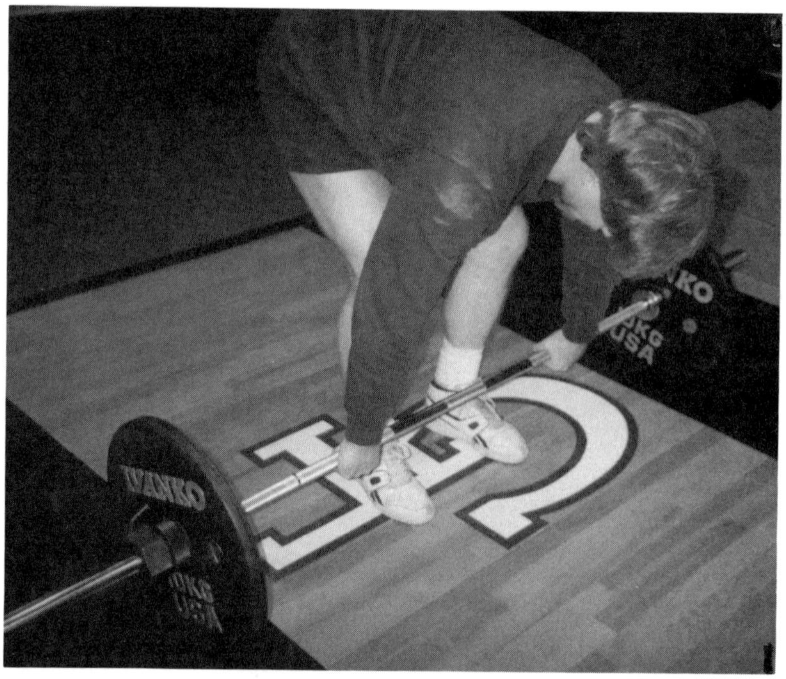

Fig. 7-8. Deadlift sequence. **(A)** Setting phase and clearance from floor; **(B)** mid-lift; **(C)** Completion. (*Figure continues.*)

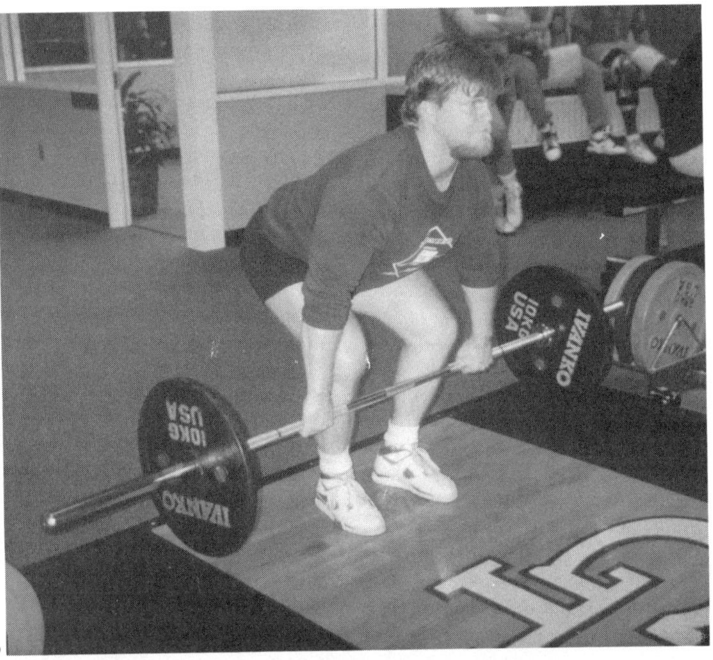

B

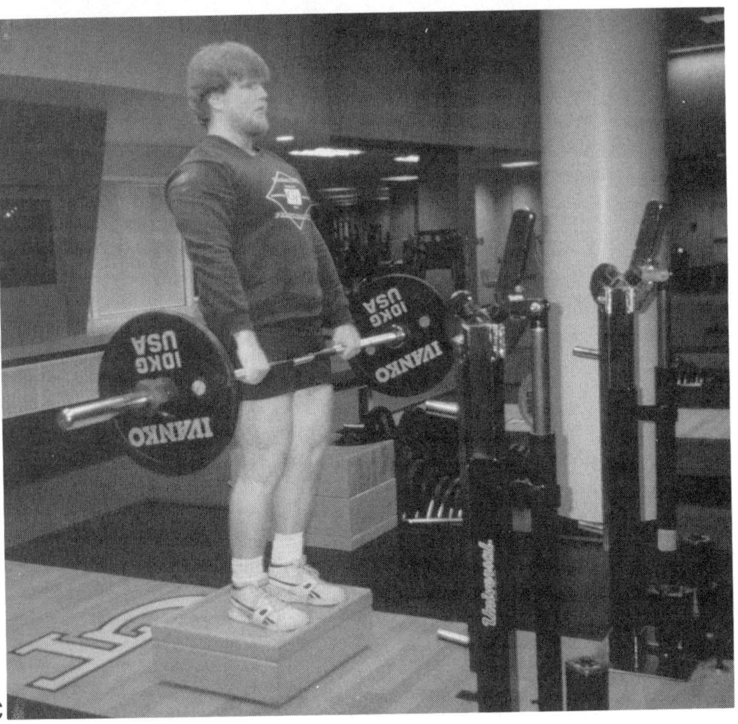

C

Fig. 7-8 *(Continued).*

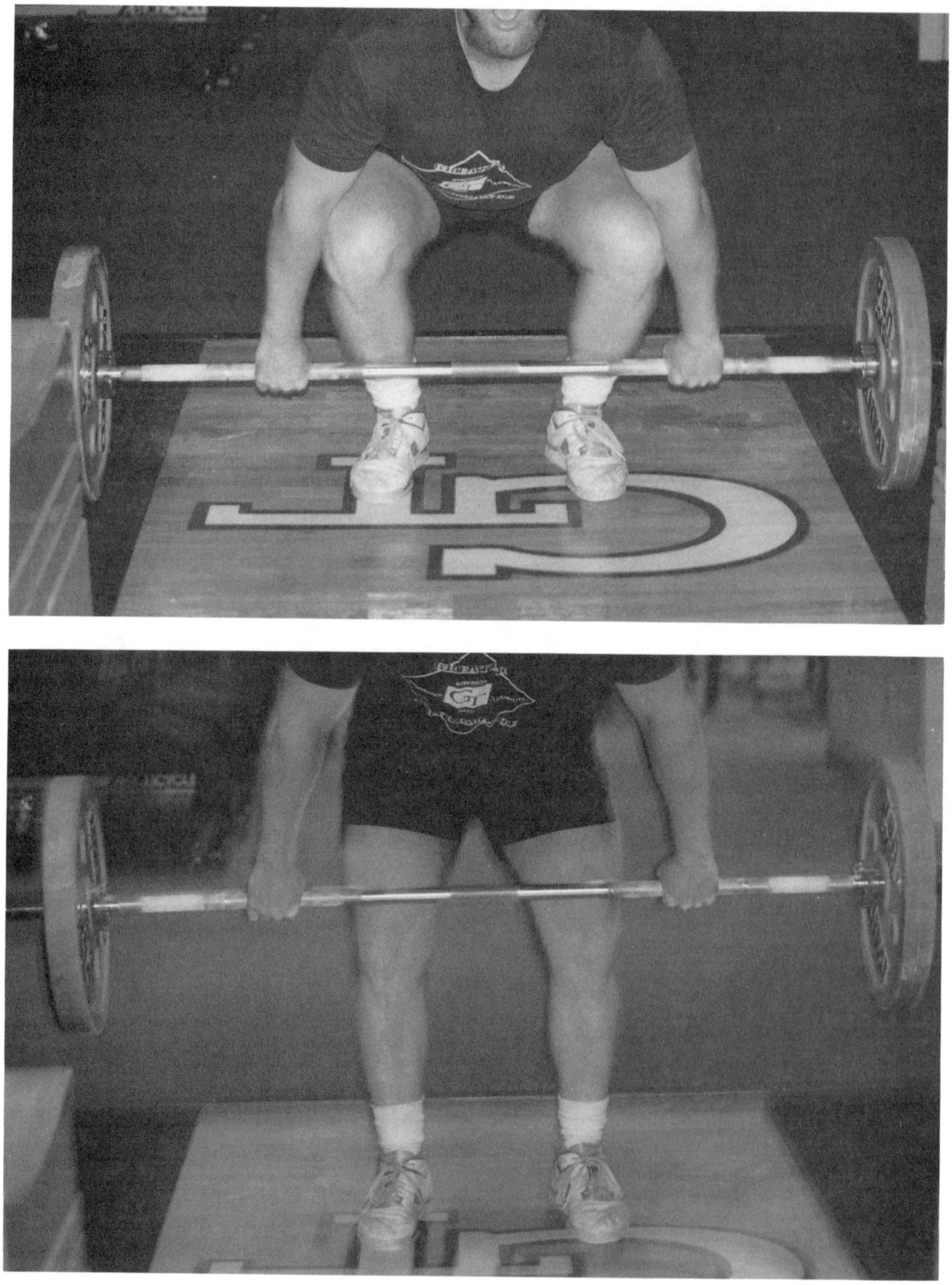

A

B

Fig. 7-9. (A–C) Power clean sequence. (*Figure continues.*)

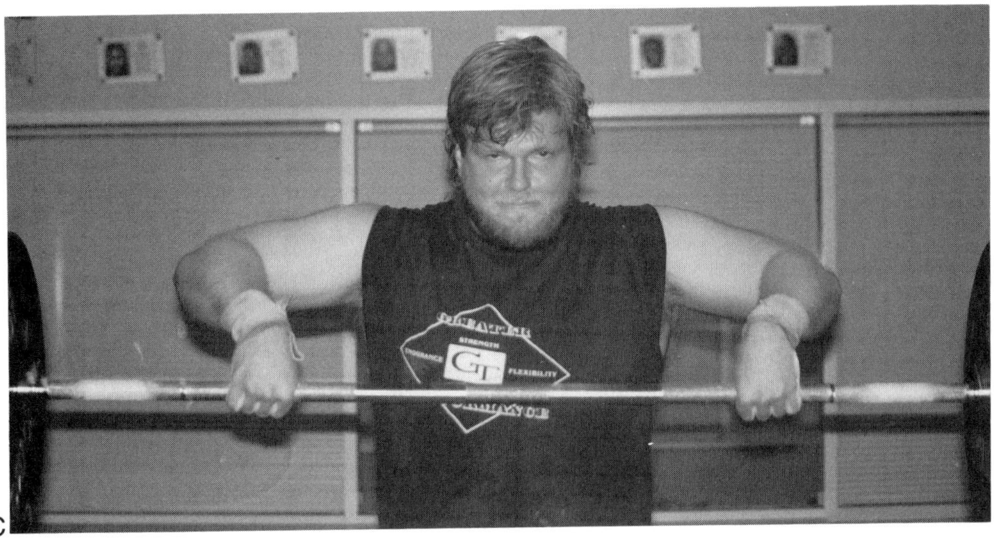

C

Fig. 7-9 *(Continued).*

forward principles. Primary to injury prevention for all physical exertional activities are the combined effects of warmup, followed immediately by the use of flexibility exercises. Warmup has been demonstrated to be effective in improving local muscle temperature and circulation, which in turn facilitates necessary viscoelasticity changes and assists in beneficial adaptations at the neuromuscular level. Flexibility exercises, preferably of static nature with 15 to 30 second holding phases, further complement the preparation of the collagen tissues for increased tensile loads. Body temperature should be increased in a gradual manner with light aerobic or simulated, light lifting movements until a light perspiration is noticed (from 5 to 15 minutes, depending on the activity, ambient temperature, and conditioning level of the individual). Appropriate, consistent breathing mechanics also serve to prevent injury to abdominal/inguinal tissues directly, as well as to secondarily prevent multiple orthopedic trauma that would result from hyperventilation or fainting during a lift. Furthermore, a thorough knowledge of correct biomechanical technique by the coaches, athletes, and spotters is critical to injury prevention. Spotters can be invaluable in providing safety to certain lifts (especially the power and Olympic lifts) and can facilitate performance through improving a lifter's confidence and concentration. Spotters should be well trained about body position and mechanics, and must remain alert and prepared throughout each phase of lifts. In addition, it is obvious that the physical layout of the gym and regular maintenance of equipment are vital to injury prevention.

Assistive devices play an important role in injury prevention as well as performance facilitation. During the squat, power clean, and Olympic style lifts it is common for lifters to wear 4-inch wide leather belts to ensure additional abdominal/lumbar stabilization. In many other lifts, particularly the bench press, the wrist/distal forearm are routinely taped for general support using cylindrical loops of adhesive, athletic tape. The knees are also wrapped with elastic, cotton wrap, which are generally used during squats and related movements. Chalk is used to maintain dry hands for a secure grip on bar lifts.

The development of lightweight, portable, and high resolution video camcorder equipment has improved one method of injury prevention that was traditionally performed with mirrors, verbal feedback, and correction. Videotaping an athlete

Table 7-7. Various Assistance Exercises Per Body Area

Chest
- Bench press with dumbbells
- Incline or decline with dumbbells or Oly bar
- Dumbbell flys
- Machine press
- Cable crossovers
- Machine flys
- Dips
- Pushups

Quadriceps
- Leg press
- Hack squat
- Front squat
- Leg extensions
- Stationary cycle
- Lunges

Hamstrings
- Machine leg curls
- Manual resistance leg curls
- Straight leg hip extensions
- Standing leg curls
- Stiff leg dead lift
- Leg press

Buttocks
- Hip and back machine
- Straight leg hip extensions
- Machine leg press
- Back squat
- Cable straight leg hip extensions

Lower back/calf
- Good mornings
- Hip and back machine
- Russian rowing
- Stiff leg dead lift
- Hyperextensions
- Gastroc/achilles/Soleus (back or lower leg)
- Machine calf raises
- Barbell calf raises
- Toe running
- Calf work on leg press

Abdomens
- Situps (weighted)
- Positional movements
- Machine work, hanging knee-ups, leg lifts
- Crunches

Abductor (inner thigh)
- Machine abductor
- Manual resistance abductor
- Cable work
- Positional movements

Abductor (outer thigh, buttocks)
- Machine abductor
- Manual resistance abductor
- Cable abductor

Neck
- 4-way neck
- Manual resistance

Anterior tibialis (front or lower leg)
- Manual resistance foot flexions
- Foot flexion on leg-pull machine

Shoulders
- Dumbbell presses (seated or standing)
- Barbell presses (front or rear)
- Forward, lateral on rear delt raises
- Machine press
- Machine lateral raises
- Cable work
- Upright row
- Shrugs (machine, dumbbell or barbell)

Latissimus dorsi (lats)
- Pulldowns (narrow or wide)
- Low cablerows
- 1-arm bentover rows
- Bentover rows (barbell or T-bar)
- Pullups (close or wide, in front or behind neck)
- Chins
- Pullover (machine, dumbbell, or EZ curl)

Biceps
- Olympic bar curls
- Dumbbell curls (seated or standing)
- Preacher curls (EZ, dumbbell, or barbell)
- Hammer curls

Forearms
- Wrist curls (regular or reverse)
- High rep grip work
- Hammer curls
- Reverse curls

Triceps
- Lying extensions
- French press
- Pushdowns (cable)
- Close grip bench press
- Dips
- Tricep kickbacks

performing a certain lift and observing the technical performance of the lift are instrumental in identifying and correcting biomechanical flaws that may predispose the athlete to injury as weight levels increase. Another use of videotaping involves the athlete viewing the lift performed by an expert before attempting it, called performance modeling.[11]

The role of proper nutrition is vital to success with strengthening programs and relates to injury prevention through alertness and concentration during lifts, adequate hydration to avoid muscle spasms that may lead to muscular or joint injury, and by the interaction of protein metabolism in repairing tissue after intense lifting bouts. Sound nutritional habits such as low dietary fat and salt, adequate calories to compensate for activity demands, appropriate hydration, and daily requirements of vitamins, minerals, fiber, and protein are all important elements that support the concept of positive adaptation to stressful muscular training.

PROGRAM DESIGN AND PRACTICAL GUIDELINES

Although subject to increasing experimental investigation, the exact combination of intensity, frequency, and type of exercise to produce optimal strength training and muscle building programs remains more often the result of personal preferences than scientific certainty.[12] Our goal, therefore, in this section is to offer guidelines for strengthening programs that are based on the empirical experience of knowledgeable weight trainers and existing scientific concepts. The basic principle of progressive overload to the muscle to stimulate strength changes is widely accepted by the scientific and health community. Recent studies also implicate the importance of the neural system and its adaptations as being paramount factors in strength increases.[13–18]

The composition of a particular individual's program is dependent on the desired physical outcome and performance objective and should be

Table 7-8. Control of Variables With Respect to Weight Training Objective

Desired Physical Outcomes	Variable Control
Cardiovascular endurance	Moderate to heavy weight, rapid contractions, the use of repeated power exercises, 6 to 10 repetitions for 3 sets, 5 to 15 seconds rest between each set and exercise.
Local muscular endurance	Light weight (10 RM), 10 to 15 repetitions, 3 sets, moderate contractions, and minimum rest interval.
Explosive power/speed	Moderate weight, 1 to 3 repetitions, rapid contractions, decreasing rest interval, 1 to 3 sets, and use of power exercises.
Muscle mass or bulk	Heavy weight, maximum number of repetitions, 2 sets, slow contractions, repeated heavy or maximum lifts, use of "flushing," or activation of the same muscle groups repeatedly to provide a prolonged flow of blood to a specific area.
Rehabilitation of injured muscles and joints	Light weights, slow contractions, 6 to 10 repetitions after initial training sessions involving no weight and 3 to 5 contractions, 3 sets, utilizing exercises that activate the supporting muscles of a joint such as those of the ankle, knee, and shoulder. Also helpful for prevention of injury to these areas.
Strength	Heavy weights (2 to 5 RM), low repetitions, slow contractions, minimum rest between sets and exercises, maximum lifts, Groves' Super-Overload Method
Strength and endurance (general body development)	Moderate weight (8 RM), 6 to 10 repetitions, moderate contractions, decreasing rest interval, 3 sets, varied exercises to activate all major muscle groups.

Abbreviation: RM, repetition maximum (see p. 149).
(Modified from Dintiman et al.,[21] with permission.)

Table 7-9. Strength Program and Exercises for Offensive and Defensive Football Linemen and Linebackers

- Monday and Thursday (muscles worked: legs/back/biceps/abs)
  - Legs
    - Squat-Cycle (Thursday—Olympic squat; Monday—power squat)
    - Cleans-cycle (Thursday—clean before squat)
      - Leg press—3 × 10–12 (perform on heavy day only)
      - Leg extensions—3 × 8–10
      - Leg curls—3 × 8–10
      - Heel raises—3 × 20 (20 reps each direction)
  - Lower back (Pick one: Straight leg deadlift—3 × 10–12)
    - or
    - (Hyperextensions—3 × 20 with weight)
  - Back work
    - Chins—3 × failure
    - Bentover rows—4 × 8–10
      - or
    - Rowing machine
  - Biceps
    - Olympic bar curls—4 × 8–10
    - Hammer curls—3 × 8–10
  - Abdominal work—150 reps, any combination
- Tuesday and Friday (muscles worked: chest/shoulders/triceps/neck)
  - Chest
    - Bench press-cycle
      - Dips—3 × 10–12 (over 12 reps, add weight)
      - Dumbbell incline—3 × 8–10 (Friday only)
      - Incline bench—4 × 6–8 (Tuesday only)
  - Shoulders
    - Military press—4 × 8–10 (perform with Olympic bar only)
      - Upright rows—3 × 8–10 (Tuesday only)
      - Shoulder shrugs—3 × 12–15 (Friday only)
      - Front raises—2 × 10–12
      - Rear flys—2 × 10–12
  - Triceps
    - Close grip bench—4 × 6–8 (Friday only)
    - Lying triceps extension—4 × 8–10
    - Pushdowns—3 × 8–10 or French press—3 × 8–10
  - Neck
    - Nautilus 4 way neck—2 × 10 (each direction)
  - Abdominal work
    - 150 reps, any combination

devised based on the principle of specificity. A review of the primary objectives with weight training programs is outlined in Table 7-8. Despite the diversity in weight training programs, the major goal of increased strength dictates regular, intense sessions from 3 to 5 times per week (dependent on specific goals), with frequent use of alternate heavy and lighter sessions and alternating days of upper body dominant training with lower body dominant sessions. Table 7-9 provides a standard model of dividing training into upper/lower body days with specific application to football. Due to physiologic recovery, the same muscle groups should not be trained intensely on consecutive days and according to Stone and O'Bryant,[19] recovery of individual body areas after intense weight training occurs in a hierarchy of fastest to slowest as follows: upper body, lower body, and low back. The implications of this hierarchy would seem to indicate that the upper body may be trained intensely up to 3 times per week, while the low back muscles should be trained no more than 2 times weekly.

Many authorities in weight training/lifting favor and emphasize the use of power cleans, squats, and bench presses as the "core" exercises in eccentric biased, strength, and hypertrophy-oriented programs.[11,19,20] These multijoint, large muscle-mass movements present a foundation for all other assistance type exercises. It is important to perform large muscle lifts first in any lifting ses-

Table 7-10. Time Allotment for Various Training Phases

Program Phase	% Time	Time (min)
Warmup		5–10
Flexibility		10–20
Power	30–45	45–60
Leg/back pulling Strength	10–12	10–20
Leg and back strength	10–20	10–20
Arm/shoulder pushing Strength	7–10	7–15
Arm/shoulder pulling Strength	7–10	7–15
Muscle endurance (Integrated into each exercise and/or one day per week of circuit training)		
Trunk and abdominal Strength	3–5	5–8
Neck strength	3–5	5–8
Rehabilitation exercises		Based on need
Warmdown		5–10

Table 7-11. Weight Standards (Body Weight + Lbs)[a]

Level	Clean	Bench Press	Dead Lift	Front Squat	Back Squat
Very poor	−25	−50	BWT + 100	BWT + 100	BWT + 250
Poor	BWT	BWT	BWT + 125	BWT + 125	BWT + 275
Average	+25	+75	BWT + 150	BWT + 150	BWT + 300
Good	+50	+100	BWT + 200	BWT + 175	BWT + 325
Excellent	+75	+150	BWT + 275	BWT + 200	BWT + 350

[a] Totals expressed in bodyweight (BWT) ± additional weight.

sion (after appropriate warmup techniques) in order to train these important groups while fresh, to provide maximal energy resources for these physically and mentally demanding lifts, and to avoid fatiguing stabilizer or synergistic muscles that may lead to faulty performance or injury.[11,19] Adequate rest periods between individual lifts are based on the type and the intensity level of the lift, with a normal range from 2 minutes to 4.5 minutes. Additional research is indicated to clarify optimal rest periods for specific free weight lifts. Total time for a single session varies from 45 to 90 minutes, again dependent on specific program goals. Although general in nature, a sample time allotment for a full body weight workout is presented in Table 7-10. It should be noted that this sample does not apply to intense weight levels, or to alternating body parts on separate days.

As a guideline for intense weight training programs using power and Olympic lifts, Table 7-11 presents weight standards for experienced lifters and/or recreational and competitive athletes. Table 7-12 quantifies the weights required for given training levels as a percentage of the 1 RM (defined as the maximum amount of weight that can correctly be lifted in one repetition). Systematic variation of lifting loads based on specific repetitions with the I RM is called cycling or periodization.[11] Varying repetitions and intensity of workouts assists in prevention of strength and pyschological plateaus (sustained periods of unchanged strength or performance of lifts).

Table 7-12. Weight Percentages

MAX.	60%	70%	75%	80%	85%	90%	95%	100%	105%
700	420	490	525	560	595	630	665	700	735
690	415	485	520	550	585	620	655	690	725
680	410	475	510	545	580	610	645	680	715
670	400	470	505	535	570	605	635	670	705
660	395	460	495	530	560	595	625	660	695
650	390	455	490	520	555	585	620	650	685
640	385	450	480	510	545	575	610	640	670
630	380	440	475	505	535	565	600	630	660
620	370	435	465	495	525	560	590	620	650
610	365	425	460	490	520	550	580	610	640
600	360	420	450	480	510	540	570	600	630
590	353	415	440	470	500	530	560	590	620
580	350	405	435	465	495	520	550	580	610
570	340	400	430	455	485	515	540	570	600
560	335	390	420	450	475	505	530	560	590
550	330	385	410	440	470	495	525	550	580
540	325	380	405	430	460	485	515	540	565

(Continued)

Table 7-12. *(continued)*

MAX.	60%	70%	75%	80%	85%	90%	95%	100%	105%
530	320	370	400	425	450	475	505	530	555
520	310	365	390	415	440	470	495	520	545
510	305	360	380	410	435	460	485	510	535
500	300	350	375	400	425	450	475	500	525
490	295	345	370	390	415	440	465	490	515
480	290	335	360	385	410	430	455	480	505
470	280	330	350	375	400	425	445	470	495
460	275	320	345	365	390	415	435	460	485
450	270	315	335	360	380	405	425	450	475
440	265	310	330	350	375	395	420	440	460
430	260	300	320	345	365	385	410	430	450
420	250	295	315	335	355	380	400	420	440
410	245	285	305	330	350	370	390	410	430
400	240	280	300	320	340	360	380	400	420
390	235	275	290	310	330	350	370	390	410
380	230	265	285	305	325	340	360	380	400
370	220	260	275	295	315	330	350	370	390
360	215	250	270	290	305	325	340	360	380
350	210	245	260	280	295	315	330	350	370
340	205	240	255	270	290	305	325	340	355
330	200	230	245	265	280	295	315	330	345
320	190	225	240	255	270	290	305	320	335
310	185	215	230	250	265	280	295	310	325
300	180	210	225	240	255	270	285	300	315
290	175	205	215	230	245	260	275	290	305
280	170	195	210	225	240	250	265	280	295
270	160	190	200	215	230	245	255	270	285
260	155	180	195	210	220	235	245	260	275
250	150	175	185	200	210	225	235	250	265
240	145	170	180	190	205	215	230	240	250
230	140	160	170	185	195	205	220	230	240
220	130	155	165	175	185	200	210	220	230
210	125	145	155	170	180	190	200	210	220
200	120	140	150	160	170	180	190	200	210
190	115	135	140	150	160	170	180	190	200
180	110	125	135	145	155	160	170	180	190
170	100	120	130	135	145	155	160	170	180
160	95	110	120	130	135	145	150	160	170
150	90	105	110	120	130	135	145	150	160
140	85	100	105	110	120	125	135	140	145
130	80	90	100	105	110	115	125	130	135
120	70	85	90	95	100	110	115	120	125
110	65	75	80	90	95	100	105	110	115
100	60	70	75	80	85	90	95	100	105

During lifting, it is important to concentrate on the specific muscle being recruited. On light load days, it is beneficial to focus on skill improvement; furthermore, as a general rule, the amount of weight lifted is secondary to efficient technique for each individual lift.[11]

CONCLUSIONS

The use of free weights provides an effective method of eccentric loading of maximal intensity for athletes and can be applied in submaximal loads for rehabilitation. Free weight training can refine many aspects of athletic performance, including injury prevention, and is both a preparatory technique and a component of plyometric training progressions. In all types of lifting and free weight programs, appropriate technique is paramount to both peak performance and injury prevention.

REFERENCES

1. Kulund DN et al: Olympic weight lifting injuries. Phys Sports Med 6:11, 1978
2. Sale DG: Neural adaptation to resistance training. Med Sci Sports Exerc, suppl. 20:S135, 1988
3. Enoka RM: Muscle Strength and its development. New Perspectives. Sports Med 6:146, 1988
4. Chandler TJ, Wilson GD, Stone MH: The effects of the squat exercise on knee stability. Med Sci Sports Exerc 21:299, 1989
5. Garhammer J: Power production by Olympic lifters. Med Sci Sports Exerc 12:54, 1980
6. Dishman RK, Gettman LR: Psychological vigor and self-perception of increased strength, abstracted. Med Sci Sports Exerc 13:73, 1981
7. Tucker LA: Weight trained experience and psychologicla well being. Percep Motor Skill 55:553, 1982
8. Tucker LA: Self concept: a function of self-perceived somatotype. J Psychol 113:123, 1983
9. Tucker LA: Effect of weight training on self concept: a profile of those influenced most. Res Q 54:389, 1983
10. Gamble JN: Strength and conditioning for the competitive athlete. p. 118. In Kulund DN (ed): The Injured Athlete. JB Lippincott, Philadelphia, 1988
11. Pasanella D, Lathrop J: Freshmen Football Manual on Strength and Conditioning. Georgia Tech Athletic Assoc., Atlanta, 1988
12. Jones DA, Rutherford CM, Parker DF: Physiological changes in skeletal muscle as a result of strength training. Q J Exp Physiol 74:233, 1989
13. Young A, Stokes M, Round JM, Edwards RHT: The effect of high resistance training on the strength and cross-sectional area of the human quadriceps. Eur J Clin Invest 13:411, 1983
14. Costill DL, Coyle EF, Fink WF et al: Adaptation in skeletal muscle following strength training. J Appl Physiol: Respir Environ Exerc Physiol 51:1437, 1979
15. Hakkinen K, Komi PV: Electromyographic changes during strength training and detraining: Med Sci Sports Exerc 15:455, 1982
16. Rutherford OM, Jones DA: The role of learning and co-ordination in strength training. Eur J Appl Physiol 55:100, 1986
17. Thorstensson A: Observations on strength training and detraining. Acta Physiol Scand 100:491, 1977
18. Dons B, Bollerup K, Bonde-Petersen F, Hancke S: The effect of weight-lifting exercise related to muscle fiber composition and cross sectional area in humans. Eur J Appl Physiol 40:95, 1979
19. Stone MH, O'Bryant HS: Weight Training: A Scientific Approach. Burgess Publishing, Minneapolis, 1984
20. O'Shea JP: Scientific Principles and Methods of Strength and Fitness. 2nd Ed. Addison-Wesley, Reading, 1976
21. Dintiman GB, Stone SS, Pennington JC et al: Discovering Lifetime Fitness: Concepts of Exercise and Weight Control. West Publishing, Minneapolis, 1984

Index

Page numbers followed by f indicate figures; those followed by t indicate tables.